EMDR in Fam

EMDR in Family Systems provides clinicians with a clear account of the EMDR process and a comprehensive, step-by-step approach to healing trauma through integrating EMDR with other therapeutic tools. The book provides a unique protocol utilizing numerous evidence-based diagnostic assessments; in-depth psychoeducation on attachment issues, Internal Family Systems therapy, and mindfulness; and Metaframeworks, a Family Systems modality, as a model to enhance EMDR. Filled with a wealth of information on the latest clinical studies on topics from the neurobiology of trauma to the effectiveness of mindfulness practices in EMDR, this book will open up a host of productive new avenues for EMDR therapists to pursue with their clients.

Diana Mille, PhD, MA, LMFT, AAMFT Approved Supervisor, EMDRIA Certified Therapist in EMDR, is the clinical director of therapeutic services at The Neurovation Center in Sandy Hook, Connecticut. She has been an adjunct and visiting professor in the Marriage and Family Therapy (MFT) graduate program at Fairfield University in Fairfield, Connecticut, and has worked as an LMFT specializing in trauma therapy at several outpatient and intensive outpatient facilities in Connecticut since 2009. She has also presented and co-presented papers at annual conferences of the International Family Therapy Association.

"This book is a major advance in the treatment of trauma. Thus, it is an indispensable tool for therapists treating clients with any trauma-related ailment. The book succeeds, brilliantly, in providing an innovative framework by which to inform the effective and efficient treatment of clients."
>—**Aníbal Torres Bernal, PhD,** associate professor and associate dean, Division of Counseling and Family Therapy, Regis University

"Dr. Mille provides a comprehensive description of the importance of healing trauma and trauma-related symptoms through EMDR therapy. As part of her proposed integrated approach, Dr. Mille makes an excellent connection between EMDR and different modalities of therapeutic intervention such as mindfulness and Internal Family Systems. Her inclusion of the Metaframeworks approach to EMDR protocol will provide a useful tool to mental health practitioners who are interested in working with families and couples."
>—**Tatiana Melendez-Rhodes, PhD, LMFT,** assistant professor and clinical coordinator, MFT Program, Central Connecticut State University

EMDR in Family Systems
An Integrated Approach to Healing Trauma

Diana Mille

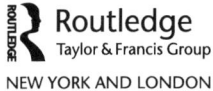

NEW YORK AND LONDON

First published 2018
by Routledge
711 Third Avenue, New York, NY 10017

and by Routledge
2 Park Square, Milton Park, Abingdon, Oxon, OX14 4RN

Routledge is an imprint of the Taylor & Francis Group, an informa business

© 2018 Taylor & Francis

The right of Diana Mille to be identified as the author of this work has been asserted by her in accordance with sections 77 and 78 of the Copyright, Designs and Patents Act 1988.

All rights reserved. No part of this book may be reprinted or reproduced or utilised in any form or by any electronic, mechanical, or other means, now known or hereafter invented, including photocopying and recording, or in any information storage or retrieval system, without permission in writing from the publishers.

Trademark notice: Product or corporate names may be trademarks or registered trademarks, and are used only for identification and explanation without intent to infringe.

Library of Congress Cataloging-in-Publication Data
Names: Mille, Diana, author.
Title: EMDR in family systems : an integrated approach to healing trauma / Diana Mille.
Description: New York : Routledge, 2018. | Includes bibliographical references and index.
Identifiers: LCCN 2017034710 | ISBN 9781138287396 (hardcover : alk. paper) | ISBN 9781138287402 (pbk. : alk. paper) | ISBN 9781315268286 (e-book)
Subjects: | MESH: Psychological Trauma—therapy | Eye Movement Desensitization Reprocessing—methods | Family Relations—psychology | Family Therapy—methods
Classification: LCC RC489.E98 | NLM WM 172.5 | DDC 616.85/210651—dc23
LC record available at https://lccn.loc.gov/2017034710

ISBN: 978-1-138-28739-6 (hbk)
ISBN: 978-1-138-28740-2 (pbk)
ISBN: 978-1-315-26828-6 (ebk)

Typeset in Galliard
by Apex CoVantage, LLC

To all those suffering from psychological trauma and the courageous individuals who have dared to embark on a difficult journey placing their trust in me to help them re-write their narrative and "make it to the other side."

To my first true love, who was also my best friend, Philippe, and many others who grapple with serious and heartbreaking mental health difficulties resulting from psychological trauma and were denied the opportunity to make that journey.

Contents

Preface viii
Acknowledgments xi

   Introduction 1

1 A World of Trauma 10

2 Quagmires in Attempting to Heal the Traumatized Brain 22

3 Eye Movement Desensitization and Reprocessing 33

4 Enhancing the EMDR Protocol: An Integrated Approach 64

5 Utilizing the Metaframeworks Perspective to Enhance the Effectiveness of EMDR in Clinical Practice 83

6 Summary, Clinical Implications and Further Research 111

Appendices 119
Index 141

Preface

> Our ability to make sense of and create meaning from memories defines how we feel about ourselves and shapes our identity we create throughout our lives.
>
> (Susan Gregory Thomas)

The Witness

The invitation to write this book came as a timely endeavor in this author's life. It has given me the opportunity to codify the latest theories and research as well as my own presentations, publications, and clinical practice in an effort to empower the use of EMDR in family systems. The intention of this book is to create a unique and integrated approach which draws from numerous supportive mechanisms including: psychoeducation; a comprehensive range of evidence-based intake, screening and diagnostic tools; attachment theory; studies surrounding the correlation between memory and trauma; Internal Family Systems; the Metaframeworks Perspective; mindfulness; and neurological techniques, all in an effort to better heal a **world of trauma** existing in both internal and external family systems.

In 2005, this author witnessed a metanoia, stemming from the Greek word *metanoiein*, signifying a transformative change of heart, *especially*, a spiritual conversion of self. Having been an art historian for over twenty years specializing in nineteenth- and twentieth-century art and architecture, concepts such as postmodernism that focus on inclusion, diversity, and integration in language and meaning were already part of my daily conscious existence in my teaching and research at Fairfield University.

I feel certain that my knowledge and use of these concepts encompassing pluralism, gender awareness, multiculturalism, and a more useful epistemology, or way of knowing, primed me for redefining myself as an LMFT, AAMFT Approved Supervisor, and an EMDRIA certified EMDR therapist embracing such integrative practices as EMDR, the Metaframeworks perspective, the Internal Family Systems model and mindfulness, to name a few, that completed my transformation to dedicate my life to healing those suffering from trauma.

One essential characteristic shared by all these modalities is that they are non-pathologizing: the client is not perceived as *diseased*.

In my personal world, however, the objective of rethinking my own narrative and having it inform my work as a therapist coincided with a series of traumas which began during my childhood, continued during my final days in the Marriage and Family Therapy (MFT) graduate program at Fairfield University in Fairfield, Connecticut, and throughout the process of getting licensed and pursuing additional credentials. "Seemingly" unaffected by my childhood trauma, I realized during my graduate studies that I was in the midst of a different trauma. It became apparent that my then spouse of 17 years was suffering from trauma, gradually becoming angry and emotionally abusive, engaging in diverse forms of risky behavior, struggling with a brief manifestation of gender dysphoria, and presenting with symptoms of an "undiagnosed" bipolar disorder that resulted in a suicide attempt, perceived by this author, and other mental health professionals as "a cry for help."

During my training to become an MFT, and my practice as an LMFT, I spent several years trying to persuade my spouse to seek help from mental health professionals. The result was minimal compliance (e.g., attending a few talk-therapy and EMDR sessions and a brief period of taking Cymbalta and other SSRIs). After 25 years of marriage, I realized that my spouse was in denial that he needed help, that his anger and risky behaviors were escalating, and that I was feeling unsafe. It was at that time that I succumbed to the dreaded but inevitable process of filing for divorce. I relocated to Savannah, Georgia, in the month of July to embark on a new life, never suspecting how brief this re-location would be. After residing for four months in Savannah, I had managed to secure a clinical position, was advising supervisees, had an adjunct LMFT teaching position in place for January 2015, and began working towards becoming an EMDRIA certified EMDR therapist.

In early November, however, my mother's health took a turn for the worse. My ex-spouse, who proclaimed that he was now attending weekly therapy sessions and under the care of a psychiatric prescriber which I was able to confirm, volunteered to help me make the arduous car journey back to Connecticut. Having no time to secure a place of residence, I rented a room temporarily in the same house where my ex-spouse, "seemingly" back in control of his life, was also renting. "What could possibly go wrong?" I thought. Well, 10 days after I arrived in Connecticut, on Thanksgiving Day to be exact, I went to celebrate the holiday with some close friends. Within an hour after arriving at their home, I began to feel physically ill and knew that "something wasn't quite right." I, therefore, immediately returned to my temporary rental quarters shared with my ex-spouse, only to discover his body hanging from a tree not more than 30 feet from the house. What could possibly go wrong, indeed!

Since we are all professionals, it is not necessary to dwell on the horrific details of what ensued in the aftermath on so many cognitive, emotional, and somatic levels. However, after witnessing this horrific event, I experienced a psychological tsunami, the flooding of childhood memories of physical, sexual, and emotional abuse from which, in Internal Family Systems (IFS) terms (see Chapter 4), my extreme manager had protected me from for so many years. However, while I sought counseling and "tried to pick up the pieces of my life," my striving manager kept pushing me forward in an effort to complete my EMDRIA certification and to accept the position of Clinical Director of Therapeutic Services at what was formerly Western Connecticut Center for Neurofeedback and Counseling, now The Neurovation Center, in Sandy Hook, Connecticut.

If it had not been for the gracious support of my therapists, mentors, supervisors, employer, colleagues, friends, and partner, all of whom will be referenced in my acknowledgements, I don't know if this witness could have kept her manager and exiles or hurt parts from becoming extreme and overwhelmed, thus threatening her very "Self."

From the very first moment that I started the process of psychologically re-writing my personal narrative, I found myself asking again and again, "how would I heal from my traumatic experiences?" One day, however, I just stopped asking; I understood. In the end, I feel blessed to have been given the opportunity to re-write both my personal and professional narrative and to continue to pursue my passion of helping others "get to the other side."

Acknowledgments

While many authors describe the process of writing a book as a solitary endeavor, I did not find this to be the case. Given the distinctive personal and professional narrative described in the Preface, there were many inspirational individuals who were figuratively "sitting next to me," inspiring my thoughts, and guiding me as I was working on this endeavor. It would take an entire publication to adequately honor these individuals whose research, courage, compassion, and support made the research and writing of this book possible. The commonly used expression, for example, that "it takes a village to raise a child," clearly reflects my personal and professional experiences and confronted me with the necessity of re-writing my narrative in the hopes of inspiring other professionals to re-write theirs with the intent of healing others.

I would like to express my deepest gratitude to the individuals who embarked on a collaborative journey with me to heal from the fragmentation of these painful memories and to bring me to a more *integrated* Self. To my extraordinarily inspired and inspiring teachers at Villa Walsh Academy in Morristown, New Jersey, words cannot express how sincerely indebted I am to them for making me see that I mattered, for giving me a voice, and for spending countless hours working with me to realize my academic potential. To the singularly gifted and compassionate professors that I had the privilege of having studied under during my undergraduate and graduate studies in both of my academic disciplines, I send my deepest appreciation. These individuals include, but are not limited to, Matthew Baigell, Tod Marder, Rosalind Krauss (who in her 2011 book *Under the Blue Cup* courageously interweaves her personal and professional journey of recovery from a brain aneurysm in 1999), Ingeborg Haug, Renee Strange, Ralph Cohen, Rona Preli, Christine Walker, and Helene Stoller. One, however, deserves a very special commendation. My gifted professor, mentor, colleague, and friend Anibal Torres Bernal guided me through some of my darkest hours, encouraging me to complete my Master's Degree in Marriage and Family Therapy. He continues his unconditional compassion and support in the present as we frequently co-present at conferences and write about our passions in the field. Thank you, my friend.

As Clinical Director of Therapeutic Services at the Neurovation Center, I would especially like to thank my clients who placed their trust in me to participate in a difficult collaborative journey towards healing their psychological traumas and my dear colleagues, a competent, dedicated, and compassionate team of clinicians, neurofeedback technicians, and support staff as I was "getting my life back." To Karen, a former Para-Educator at Sandy Hook School and now a gifted neurofeedback technician and a great writer, I offer my deepest appreciation for having the courage to come forward and tell her story "Not All the Victims Die" (see Appendix 1). To Melissa, another great mind and senior neurofeedback technician, and "alter ego," I am deeply indebted for literally "taking my hand" and "walking me through" the most potent difficulties for this author. Her creativity in helping me to bring to life my personalized mandala, a cosmic diagram, and *integrated* structure (see Introduction) as well as her unprecedented technical skills and patience in creating and placing my diagrams and other compensatory information will be forever cherished.

To my friend Jeffrey Schutz, owner and Executive Director of The Neurovation Center, and the most accomplished, compassionate, professional, and courageous colleague and clinician I have ever known, I offer my deepest gratitude for literally "saving my professional life," by hiring and re-hiring me after the most traumatic moments that I witnessed in my life. Although suffering the horrific loss of his 16-year-old son Joel in February, 2016, Jeff and his business partner and wife, Laurie, continued to believe in me and my qualifications and dedication to help heal a traumatized community and provided me with every professional and personal tool that I requested to accomplish this task.

Along with Jeff, I am also gratefully indebted to Lindsay K. Higdon, Clinical Director of Neurofeedback Services and Senior QEEG Analyst and Diplomat. They provided me with a well-crafted and clearly articulated synthesis of the healing potential of combining neurofeedback and EMDR (see Appendix 4). To Elizabeth Graber, editor at Routledge: Taylor & Francis Group, who reached out to me to write this book and took me through the initial steps of codifying the intent of my book, obtaining the initial readers and finalizing the agreement with the publisher, I offer my sincerest gratitude. To my publisher, George Zimmer, editorial assistant, Nina Guttapalle, and project manager, Holly González Smithson at Apex CoVantage, I extend my deepest appreciation for guiding me through a difficult process with an endless sense of commitment, support, flexibility, and a unique and encouraging graceful demeanor.

I would like to express my sincerest debt to dedicated and courageous researchers, professors, and mental health psychiatrists and clinicians such as Bessel van der Kolk, Florence W. Kaslow, Louise Maxfield, Elan Shapiro, Peter A. Levine, Richard C. Schwartz, Douglas C. Breunlin, Betty Mac Kune-Karrer, William M. Pinsof, Ralph Cohen, Daniel J. Siegel, Ronald D. Siegel, Jon Kabat-Zinn, Stephen W. Porges, Jeremy Holmes, Christopher K. Germer, Paul R. Fulton, Monica McGoldrick, and John Bowlby, among many others mentioned throughout my book, who were willing to "step out of the box" to explore many diverse protocols to enhance EMDR in the healing of psychological trauma in family systems. This book would not be possible without their contributions.

It is to Francine Schapiro, however, that we all must offer our admiration and thanks for her fortuitous discoveries made during a traumatic period in her life which resulted one day in 1987 when taking a "simple walk in the park," and her subsequent intense and selfless work to codify the evidence-based EMDR protocol, that has been used for many decades to heal those suffering from diverse, multileveled, and multidimensional traumas.

To my long-time friends Conrad, Chuck, Betsy, Cathy, Dave, Russ, Amy, Alla, Deborah, Dave, Tom, Buda, Trish, Victor, Maryann, Marcy, Mimi, Bill, Bob, Claude, and my long-term friend and colleague Robin, who consistently watched over me every step of the way during my adult traumatic experiences, offering unconditional support and love, I would like to express my profound gratitude for helping me to "take the baby steps" necessary to reclaim my life, my voice, and my passion to help others.

No words can express my debt to my partner Rick, a dedicated professor, scholar, and author of nine books and many articles, for his unconditional generosity of spirit in reading my draft with a discerning eye, for always being on the "lookout" for unique and relevant materials that I might add to my manuscript, for his constant and enthusiastic support, and for the inordinate amount of patience that he demonstrated in calming an author often overwhelmed by a taxing clinical, presenting, and publishing schedule. Like my high school teachers mentioned above, he continually validated my worth, encouraged the importance of keeping my voice, and reminded me of the uniqueness that I could bring to *the world of trauma* which needed to be brought to fruition to help other like-minded researchers and clinicians to continue their journey to help those in pain.

Introduction

> I pray you are what waits to break back into the world.
> (Tracy K. Smith, 2011)

According to the National Center for PTSD approximately 8 million adults suffer from Post-Traumatic Stress Disorder (PTSD) in a given year, which is listed under the category of Trauma-and Stress-related Disorders in the DSMV. This suggests that many who experience traumatic events are likely to suffer from posttraumatic stress disorder, an anxiety-related disorder.

Trauma is also at the root of the vast majority of mental health diagnoses. We may diagnose Generalized Anxiety Disorder, but trauma is often the underlying cause. We may diagnose Major Depression, but trauma again is often the real cause. Even with attention-deficit hyperactivity disorder (ADHD), we have found that trauma frequently is the prime contributor to the symptoms we use to diagnose focus problems.

In her 2017 article "Power, Agency, and Resilience after Trauma," Ruth C. Neustifter recognizes, "Clinical definitions of trauma often focus on diagnostic criteria related to symptoms of ongoing distress. *Merriam Webster Dictionary (2017)* defines it as '. . . a disordered psychic or behavioral state resulting from severe mental or emotional stress or physical injury,' or an 'emotional upset'" (p. 11).

The word *trauma* in the Greek language originally meant "wound" in the physical sense, but we all know that this has morphed in our field to signify a psychological state that describes a condition in which the person has experienced a difficult event that has wounded the psyche. Psychological trauma is a type of damage to the psyche that occurs as a result of an overwhelming, distressing event. Furthermore, trauma also has etiological roots in the Greek word "injury," the result of an overwhelming amount of stress, the effects of which can be delayed by a week, days, years, or even decades, but that can eventually catch up with one and prove debilitating.

Psychological trauma often manifests as a cluster of symptoms, adaptations, and reactions that interfere with the functioning of an individual who has experienced extreme suffering, resulting from serious bodily harm, physical abuse/assault, sexual and emotional abuse, neglect, domestic violence, being the victim of an alcoholic parent, experiencing a life-threatening disease, bullying, witnessing or surviving an accident, natural disaster, mass violence, suicide, terrorism, or combat.

Psychological trauma is something that overwhelms the individual from an emotional, cognitive, and somatic perspective and affects their ability to cope, function, and communicate on personal and professional levels. It has three main components—it was unexpected, the individual or individuals were unprepared, and there was nothing they could do to prevent it from happening, singularly or repeatedly.

The impact of trauma is powerful and multidimensional in terms of invading and fragmenting the self-structure and its inter-personal connections. The whole of the person is "wounded" or "injured" since trauma affects many dimensions of behavioral and physical functioning. The effects of trauma, for example, create symptoms of anxiety, depression, dissociation, low self-esteem, emotional detachment, mood swings, despair, panic attacks, and self-destructive tendencies, to name a few. On a physical level, trauma can present with nightmares, insomnia, eating disorders, hallucinations, difficulties concentrating, muscle pain, and fatigue, among other symptoms. On a more relational level, trauma causes changes in worldview (e.g., loss of spirituality, uncertainty, and disorganization of 'self'), beliefs about human nature, patterns of intimacy, interpersonal relationships, and conceptions of oneself and personal identity.

Power and resilience also play a critical role in defining the traumatic experience. As Neustifter explains,

> Once trauma has been identified questions of power often arise. The survivors that I have interviewed and spoken with have almost universally noted a situation, series of situations, or an ongoing situation in which they have felt powerlessness or much less powerful than the oppressive or harming person, people, or situations.
>
> (p. 11)

As Neustifter notes about resiliency, which is "the process of adapting well in the face of adversity, trauma, tragedy, threats or significant sources of stress," client interviews suggest that "resilience might be defined as the ability to reclaim our lives and ourselves after trauma, and to redefine success for ourselves, and to move toward it" (p. 11). Neustifter recognizes that "healthy and positive acclimatization and the reduction of distress over symptoms [also] becomes a frequent [and necessary] goal" in the treatment of trauma (p. 11).

In his seminal 2015 book *Trauma and Memory: Brain and Body in a Search for the Living Past*, Peter Levine explains, "In contrast to 'ordinary' memories (both good and bad), which are mutable and dynamically changing over time, traumatic memories are fixed and static. They are imprints (engrams) from past overwhelming experiences, deep impressions carved into the sufferer's brain, body and psyche" (p. 7). As Levine continues, "In sharp contrast to gratifying or even troublesome memories, which can generally be formed and revised as coherent narratives, 'traumatic memories' tend to arise as fragmented splinters of inchoate and indigestible sensations, emotions, images, smells, tastes, thoughts and so on" (p. 7). Extreme fragmentation of the self-structure leads to an adverse impact on inter-personal behaviors and functioning, namely, an absence of the ability to connect. This disconnect may be manifested in the following symptom clusters: dissociation—a wide array of experiences from mild detachment from immediate surroundings to more severe detachment from physical and emotional experience—alienation, mistrust, isolation, anhedonia, impulsiveness, impaired sensuality, shame, fear, anger, inability to relax or self-soothe, inappropriate personal boundaries, and self-defeating behaviors (Wilson and Keane, 2004; see Chapters 3 and 4 in this volume).

In addition, traumatic memories affect how we experience our present and our future from a neurobiological approach. In his 2006 essay "An Integrated Neurobiology Approach to Psychotherapy," Daniel J. Siegel notes, "memory shapes how we experience the present and how we anticipate the future, readying us in the present moment for what comes next based on what we've experienced in the past" (p. 252). As Siegel further explains, "One proposal about trauma's effects on memory is that it may transiently block the integrative function of the hippocampus in memory integration. With massive stress hormone secretion or amygdala discharge in response to an overwhelming event, the hippocampus may be shut down temporarily" (p. 253). In the end, as Siegel suggests, "The resultant neural configuration of blocked hippocampal processing, when reactivated [in the present], can present itself as free-floating, unassembled elements of perception, bodily sensation, emotion, and behavioral response, without the internal sense that something is coming from the past" (p. 253). The significance of Siegel's insights will be further referenced throughout this book.

I recognize that my readers are mental health professionals and that they know that trauma is a global epidemic. We all know that trauma constitutes one of the greatest crises facing the mental health field. Its effects are felt simultaneously on the individual as well as on global and systemic levels. In the United States alone, 3.6% of the population suffers from trauma. In a 2013 World Health Organization (WHO) study of 21 countries, more than 10% of respondents reported witnessing violence (21.8%), or experiencing interpersonal violence (18.85 %), accidents (17.7%), exposure to war (16.2%), or trauma to a loved one (12.5%) (WHO/Geneva, 2013). An estimated 3.6% of the world's population has suffered from post-traumatic stress disorder (PTSD) in previous wars (WHO/GENEVA, 2013); additional statistics on specific traumas as well as those that address multicultural and gender identity will be provided in Chapter 1.

Although trauma has been identified by many researchers as the fifth most common psychiatric disorder and is said to be the number one cause of suicide, in the opinion of this author, the onerous statistics and my clinical experiences, as well as those of my colleagues, inform us that there remains an inherent absence of effective systems of *integrated* care for the treatment of trauma in internal and external family systems.

As most of my readers are aware, the concept behind Eye Movement Desensitization and Reprocessing (EMDR) did not originate from any theoretical underpinnings or from scholarly research, but was discovered by Francine Shapiro in 1987 during "a walk in the park." Dr. Shapiro was experiencing the kind of anxiety that often accompanies trying to launch a doctoral dissertation along with the anxiety of having been diagnosed with cancer which, although successfully removed, carried the potential to rear its ugly head in the years to come, as indicated by the medical professionals who treated her. It was during this unsettling period in her life that Shapiro observed her bilaterally-generated eye movements triggered by the moving patterns of lights in nature. This observation left Shapiro with feeling a calm that quelled her anxious thoughts. By 1991, EMDR therapy was first defined and then codified by Shapiro into an integrated model embracing aspects of psychodynamic, neurobiological, experiential, behavioral, cognitive, and body-based therapies within an elegantly structured protocol.

Shapiro's protocol includes an eight-phase modality: history-taking; preparation; assessment; desensitization; installation; body scan; closure; and reevaluation; as well as a three-pronged strategy for integrating information in the brain, which alleviates past experiences, current triggers, and potential future challenges. In addition, Shapiro formulated an adaptive information-processing theory, the framework of EMDR, which addresses trauma-related symptoms by processing components of negative memories and associating them with more adaptive behaviors, emotions, and information.

In her 2007 article "EMDR, Adaptive Information Processing and Case Conceptualization," Shapiro explains, "In its 20-[now 30] year history, it [EMDR] has evolved from a simple technique into an integrative psychotherapy approach with a theoretical model that emphasizes the brain's information processing system and memories in disturbing experiences as the basis of pathology" (p. 3).

Over the past 15 years, evidence-based research and over 30 randomized clinical trials demonstrate that EMDR is extremely effective in reducing trauma and trauma-related symptoms such as depression and anxiety. More importantly, EMDR has been recognized as the first line of treatment for trauma by the World Health Organization; the American Psychiatric Association; the U.S. Department of Veterans' Affairs; the U.S. Department of Defense in the United Kingdom; the Department of Health; and the International Society of Traumatic Stress Studies. In 2010, EMDR was reviewed and included in the Substance Abuse and Mental Health Services Administration's National Registry of Evidence-based Programs and Practices (see Chapter 1).

Although we have numerous evidence-based studies that recognize EMDR as the first line of treatment for healing trauma, and while the use of the EMDR protocol has grown exponentially and its growth is not likely to subside in the near future, the continued existence of a World of Trauma, and the statistics that support this tragedy, demand a more meaningful, theoretical, and contemporary definition and understanding of trauma as well as more comprehensive, effective, and diverse integrated approaches to heal those suffering from the toxic memories of trauma. As American anthropologist Clifford Geertz (1973) so aptly explains in his book *Religion as a Cultural System*,

> Although it is notorious that definitions establish nothing, in themselves they do, if they are carefully enough constructed, provide a useful orientation, or reorientation, of thought, such that an extended unpacking of them can be an effective way of developing and controlling a novel line of inquiry.
> (p. 90)

Furthermore, EMDR is a critical centerpiece and, in part, a neurological protocol (see Chapter 3) that, when used with family systems models such as the Internal Family Systems therapy model and the Metaframeworks perspective (see Chapters 4 and 5), is crucial to healing trauma in both internal and external family systems.

There are other neurological treatments, such as neurofeedback (see Appendix 4), Electroconvulsive Therapy (ECT) (in which small electric currents are passed through the brain which trigger a brief seizure, which may cause changes in the chemistry of the brain), and Tapping/energy psychology (EFT) (that is arguably based on the concept of neuroplasticity). Most of these approaches, with the exception of neurofeedback, however, are in my opinion more limited given the controversy surrounding their efficacy and their lack of integration, which limits their relevance given the systemic focus of this book (see Chapter 3). Much of the same could be said for acupuncture, which the preponderance of scientific studies has found wanting (Interlandi, 2016).

Other more substantial talk therapy models such as Cognitive Behavioral Theory (CBT), often touted as another therapy for treating trauma with evidence-based research to support it, is already incorporated into EMDR's protocol and, as such, in my opinion, has more potency within the EMDR framework than when being utilized as a "stand-alone" therapy (see Chapter 3).

The unique purpose and scope of this book is to place EMDR into a larger therapeutic context by taking a more holistic approach, since we can seldom employ "pure" treatment modalities for healing trauma. This integrated focus is necessary to comprehend the mechanisms underlying trauma and to offer EMDR trauma clinicians a more comprehensive package for healing trauma, especially given that EMDR itself is an *integrated* approach. This method begins by providing more substantial psychoeducation on trauma and EMDR in an effort to enhance trust and empower my clients to make more informed choices regarding their treatment. For those mental health professionals who tend to advocate for more "purist" approaches regarding therapy and fear the complexity of an integrated approach, I would urge them to consider that an integrated psyche is achieved through integrated treatment modalities.

Within this holistic approach, treatment includes the identification and exploration of my clients' secure and insecure attachment styles and subsequent relationship patterns. As we all know, from the dedicated work of John Bowlby and many others, attachment styles, formulated during the first years of a child's life, often predict later behavioral trends, social adjustment skills, and concepts around self-image within both their internal and external family systems (see Chapter 4).

The all-important use of the genogram is also crucial in my understanding of what takes place in the "meaning making" of those suffering from trauma. A comprehensive and powerful joining tool, the genogram allows me to collect and map invaluable family history and structure, mental health diagnoses, epigenetics, traumas, medical problems, and inter-relational patterns across multiple generations in a rapid and easily interpreted format (see Chapter 4). Utilizing a comprehensive and *integrated* range of general and trauma-specific evidence-based intakes, screening and diagnostic tools, as well as a uniquely designed assessment, the "EMDR case conceptualization," an in-depth inquiry to target and understand the typology of the trauma, (which will be addressed in Chapter 4) promotes a more informed hypothesis.

Stephen W. Porges' polyvagal theory has also inspired my *integrated* approach with its ground-breaking understanding of how emotions, attachment, communication, and self-regulation factor into the treatment of trauma (see Chapters 3 and 4). Similarly, enhancing self-regulation with the practice of mindfulness is an effective antidote to psychological distress. The mind becomes corrupted when negative and fearful emotions enter our unconscious or conscious states. Mindfulness works in tandem with the Internal Family Systems (IFS) model as well as with EMDR's phase of stabilization (see Chapter 4). As such, it can promote safety and self-regulation by allowing those suffering from trauma to self-soothe, stay safe, increase self-confidence, and promote reintegration of memory and somatic experiences. Jon Kabat-Zinn defines mindfulness in his book *Wherever You Go, There You Are: Meditation in Everyday Life* (2005) as, "paying attention in a particular way on purpose in the present moment, and nonjudgmentally" (p. 16). It follows that if one can remain in the present moment, still and observing and ready to receive without being judgmental, one can distance oneself from negative emotions, fears, and suffering, thus decreasing stress, rumination, and reactivity, products of traumatic memories (see Chapter 4). Other visual and experiential techniques to promote safety among our traumatized internal and external family systems such as the Healing Light Visualization, Progressive Muscle Relaxation Technique and Yoga, to name a few, will also be considered (see Chapter 4).

As Clinical Director of Therapeutic Services at The Neurovation Center in Sandy Hook, Connecticut, and as an EMDRIA certified EMDR therapist, I recognize the necessity and practicality of mastering such tools given the obvious fact that individual experiences often lead to an internal sense of "self" that profoundly impacts clients' ability to relate to others in a functional and effective capacity. The unfortunate and obvious conclusion is that past traumas always impair the current internal and external systems. As a result, it has been my goal as an author to enhance EMDR in my clinical practice by integrating it with a family systems modality such as the Metaframeworks perspective, which takes a common factors approach to looking at various parameters of the human systems, the constraints in the biopsychosocial systems and within the individual metaframeworks or domains, thus serving as a critical assessment tool (see Chapter 4) as well as a timely therapeutic systemic protocol (see Chapter 5) in my research and clinical practice. However, the Metaframeworks perspective is not only integrated in its elegant assessment qualities, but is also integrated as a result of its user-friendly and comprehensive blueprint for hypothesizing, planning, giving feedback, and conversing to better address traumas and many other mental health diagnoses in both the internal/individual and external/couple subsystem.

While researchers have often made efforts to integrate EMDR with family systems therapies such as Structural Family Therapy; Experiential Therapy; Contextual Therapy; Bowen Family Therapy; and Integrative Family Therapy, to name a few, as far as I am aware, the integration of a partially neurological protocol such as EMDR with the Metaframeworks perspective has not been considered in the extant literature. As such, I believe that this author's understanding of *hermeneutics* (theory of interpretation) offers a fresh perspective that provides a broader understanding of the complexity of the human condition and a way to find order and healing within such complexity.

As a former art historian, passionate about the integrative aspect of postmodernism, I feel strongly that a "mandala" serves us as the best visual metaphor for the integrated purpose and the scope of this book (Figure 0.1).

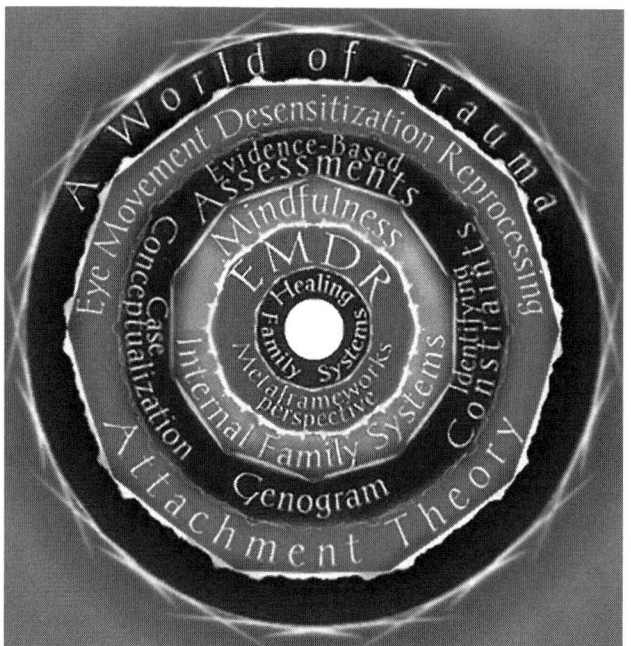

Figure 0.1 Mandala

The word *mandala* stems from the classical Indian language Sanskrit. Loosely translated to mean "a sacred circle," it represents wholeness; it is a cosmic diagram. Specifically, a mandala is an *integrated* structure, a view of the world, organized around a unifying center. While long revered by some Eastern religions, the mandala has begun to emerge in Western and other secular cultures and offers the potential for a change in how we view ourselves given its ability to nurture our development towards enlightenment and bring about inner peace.

In his book *Man and His Symbols* (1964), Carl Jung saw the mandala as both a symbol of safety and as a reconciliation of dysfunctional elements into a greater wholeness. As Jung noted, "The mandala serves a conservative purpose—namely to restore a previously existing order. But it also serves the creative purpose of giving expression and form to something that does not yet exist, something new and unique" (p. 247). The synthesis of the mandala as a symbol of rediscovering life, meaning, and order resonates with many of us. As my readers will witness throughout this book, the visual, theoretical, and practical implications of the *integration* of EMDR unfold as we move from the outermost circle, symbolizing a World of Trauma, inwards through ever more specific therapeutic inquires until we arrive at our destination: a healthy "self" in family systems (meant to reference both an internal/individual and external/couple subsystem) that is free of the destructive effects of trauma.

As mental health professionals, most of us are familiar with the quagmires that might thwart our attempt to heal the traumatized brain, including such controversial research topics as: the inadequate presence of trauma in the DSM-V; the inefficacy of talk therapy alone; and the lack of effective medications to address trauma symptomology, all of which will be addressed by the author (see Chapter 2). As the reader will see, these approaches simply do not speak to the toxic repetitive memories, difficulties self-regulating, intense negative emotions, and somatic complaints that keep our clients missing a collaborating and liberating journey and remaining, in fact, "lost in translation."

I hope this book will be helpful for clinicians, researchers, instructors, and theorists in our field as an essential psychoeducational guide in preparing our traumatized population to make a more informed choice in seeking quality treatment, thus, "getting their lives back," with the Sandy Hook school shooting on December 14, 2012, as one of the most disturbing cases in point (see Appendix 1). In the aftermath of the shooting, for example, instead of being informed of how to receive effective trauma treatment, my present clients, e.g., teachers, para-educators, and staff, tell me that they were asked innocuous questions such as "What do you want?" "Do you want to come in and talk?" "What special meals would you like us to provide you with?" and "Would you like to use the massage chairs we have supplied?" Furthermore, their being largely neglected in the discussions of the planning of the new school and what could be done to minimize their pain as they went back to "the scene of the crime" and their being left with little help addressing their financial needs, explains why many who experienced "the day" are just now seeking trauma therapy four years later.

It is my most fervent wish that this book will inspire other like-minded professionals to continue to explore the integration of EMDR and other theoretical and neurobiological techniques with family systems models such as the Metaframeworks perspective as well as to explore how multicultural and gender issues factor into the systems paradigm. I am certain all my readers will agree that there is a need for more diverse, random, double-blind quantitative studies that attend to validity and reliability when investigating various neurobiological therapies—all of them ideally nonpathologizing—that will help support the efficacy of an integrated approach such as EMDR to healing trauma in family systems (see Chapter 6). Then we can all fulfill our duty to be the change we want to see in the world.

References

Geertz, C. (1973). "Religion as a Cultural System." *The Interpretation of Cultures*. New York: Basic Books, 87–125.

Interlandi, J. (2016). "Research Casts Doubt on the Value of Acupuncture." *Scientific American*. www.scientificamerican.com/article/research-casts-doubt-on-the-value-of-acupunture/ Accessed September 7, 2016.

Jung, C.G. (1964). *Man and His Symbols*. London: Aldus Books.

Kabat-Zinn, J. (2005). *Wherever You Go, There You Are: Meditation in Everyday Life*. New York: Hachette Books.

Levine, P.A. (2015). *Trauma and Memory: Brain and Body in a Search for a Living Past*. Berkeley, CA: North Atlantic Books.

Neustifter, R.C. (2017). "Power, Agency, and Resilience after Trauma." *Family Therapy Magazine (ftm)*, 16(1), 8–11.

Shapiro, F. (2007). "Adaptive Information Processing, and Case Conceptualization." *Journal of EMDR Practice and Research*, 1(2), 68–87.

Siegel, D.J. (2006). "An Interpersonal Neurobiology Approach to Psychotherapy." *Psychiatric Annuals*, 36(4), 248–256.

Smith, T.K. (2011). *Life on Mars: Poems*. Minneapolis: Graywolf Press, 33.

WHO Media Centre. (2013). "WHO Releases Guidance on Mental Health Care after Trauma." www.who.int/mediacentre/news/releases/2013/trauma_mental_health_20130806/en/ Accessed on September 13, 2016.

Wilson, J.P., & Keane, T.M. (2004). *Assessing Psychological Trauma and PTSD*. New York: Guilford Press.

1 A World of Trauma

With my Introduction having provided my readers with a brief overview of psychological trauma including a concise definition of psychological trauma, a cursory discussion of its impact on self-structure and implications for interpersonal relationships, and the existence of staggering statistics in support, this chapter takes a more in-depth and inclusive look at the conceptual and theoretical framework of trauma (whether it is a *large T* trauma, *small t* trauma, or complex trauma), and introduces systemic implications to be continued in later chapters. It addresses Posttraumatic Stress Disorder (PTSD), the comorbidity of trauma and other mental health diagnoses, and provides supporting statistics.

Much to my surprise, and probably to the surprise of my readers, the foundations for the concepts of trauma, memory, and their implications utilized in my book were actually formulated at the end of the nineteenth century. These include intense emotions, problematic behaviors, and intense negative cognitions. As Peter A. Levine points out in his recent book *Trauma and Memory: Brain and Body in a Search for the Living Past*, the first publication "on what we now would call PTSD, *L'automatisme psychologique*," was written by Pierre Janet in 1889, "in which he argued that trauma is held in procedural memory—in automatic actions and reactions, sensations and attitudes, and that trauma is replayed and reenacted as visceral sensations (anxiety and panic), body movements, or visual images (nightmares and flashbacks)" (Levine, 2015, p. xi). As Levine continues, "Janet put the issue of memory front and center in dealing with trauma: An event only becomes a trauma when overwhelming emotions interfere with proper memory processing" (2013, p. xi).

In Levine's chapter, "Lay of the Land," he eloquently explains:

> Throughout the ages people have been tormented by memories that have filled them with fright and horror, with feelings of helplessness, rage, hatred, and revenge, and with a plaguing sense of irreparable loss. In ancient literature, such as the epic tragedies of the Greeks, Sumerians, and Egyptians, as well as hundreds of contemporary books on trauma, nightly newscasts, and celebrity confessionals, trauma has been and continues to be at the epicenter of human experience.
>
> (2013, p. xix)

As we can see, the ideas that Janet formulated about trauma in 1889 predict the perspective on psychological trauma briefly considered in my Introduction. These include: its overwhelming symptoms; the adaptations and reactions that interfere with the emotional, cognitive, and somatic functioning of the individual; and the inability of the individual to prevent and cope with the trauma.

So why in the twenty-first century is this author still asking why trauma is "under-recognized, under-diagnosed, and under-treated" on many clinical levels? One study, conducted at the "micro" or agency level in Connecticut, provides a particularly eye-opening description of the current functioning of trauma services. This study identified trauma as being prevalent across 19 agencies with 56% of clients carrying a written diagnosis directly related to traumatic experiences as well as limited evidence of the utilization of best practices across these agencies such as mandatory, formal screening and assessing; direct questioning and a written self-report; spontaneous self-disclosure and records; and trauma-specific interventions.

Furthermore, this study conducted at the agency level revealed the majority of agencies offering no specific trauma services, cross-referral mechanisms, and trauma-related supervision and education of its counselors. One service, however, that was offered at the agency level was safety planning for victims of domestic and sexual abuse (Hanson et al., 2002).

Since this study raised endless questions for me regarding the inefficacy of diagnosing and treating trauma at the agency level, it enhanced my determination and commitment to explore this enigma from the very beginning of my trauma practice and research, beginning in 2009. After many years of practice, instructing, and research, Chapter 4 exists as the culmination of my efforts to offer a more comprehensive range of inclusive and accessible general and trauma-specific evidence-based intakes and screening and diagnostic tools. Chapter 4 also lobbies for the inclusion of other potent assessments including: EMDR case conceptualization; the genogram; and the biopsychosocial continuum offered by the Metaframeworks perspective, a perspective based on identifying constraints that are functions of six core domains of organization, development, sequences, multicultural contexts, gender, and the mind.

While I addressed the impact of trauma on self-structure in my Introduction, it is important to consider an individual's subjective experience in determining the extent to which the damage to the self- structure will take place. It is often the case that it is not the event that determines whether something is traumatic to someone, but their experience of the event which is often dependent on the severity of the event, the individual's personal history, the broader meaning that the event represents for the individual, the coping skills, values and beliefs of the individual, and the support, personal and professional, that they receive from those around them.

However, according to Peter Levine in his 2010 book *In an Unspoken Voice: How the Body Releases Trauma and Restores Goodness*, "Until the core *physical* experience—feeling scared stiff, frozen in fear or collapsing and going numb— unwinds and transforms, one remains stuck, a captive of one's own entwined fear and helplessness. These sensations of paralysis or collapse seem intolerable, utterly unacceptable; they terrify and threaten to entrap and defeat us" (pp. 73–74; emphasis mine). Luckily, however,

> the human nervous system is designed and attuned both to receive and to offer a regulating influence to another person. Thankfully biology is on our side. This transference of succor, our mammalian birthright, is fostered by the therapeutic tone and working alliance you create by tuning in to your client's sensibilities.
>
> (p. 74)

Furthermore, the extreme fragmentation of the self-structure leads to an adverse impact on interpersonal behaviors and functioning, which is often described as a loss of connection. The impact on interpersonal relationships is manifested through the following symptom clusters: alienation, mistrust, anhedonia, impulsiveness, impaired sensuality, anger, inability to relax, inappropriate personal boundaries, and self-defeating behaviors (Wilson and Keane, 2004). According to Judith Lewis Herman (1992), "In survivors of childhood abuse [and in particular physical and sexual child abuse], these disturbances in relationship are further amplified" (p. 385). As Herman continues, "All the structures of the self—the image of the body, the internalized images of others, and the values and ideals that lend a sense of coherence and purpose—are invaded and systematically broken down" (p. 385). More importantly, Herman recognizes that "these disturbances are described most fully in patients with borderline personality disorder, the majority of whom have extensive histories of childhood abuse" (p. 385; see study conducted by Herman et al., 1989).

Complex Trauma

Herman's insights demonstrate the existence of complex trauma/DESNOS (Disorders of Extreme Stress Not Otherwise Specified), a syndrome that was initially considered, but never included in either the DSM-IV or the DSM-V. "The current psychiatric diagnostic system," according to the National Child Traumatic Stress Network, "does not have an adequate category to capture the full range of difficulties that traumatized children experience. Although the narrowly defined PTSD diagnosis is often used, it rarely captures the extent of the developmental impact of multiple and chronic trauma exposure" (p. 6).

Herman defines a complex post-traumatic syndrome as existing in survivors where "prolonged, repeated victimization" exists and includes prolonged and consecutive childhood abuse at an early age, which involves a betrayal of trust and coercive control in primary relationships. The National Child Traumatic Stress Network (NCTSN) reinforces Herman's insights:

> The term complex trauma describes the dual problem of children's exposure to traumatic events and the impact of this exposure on immediate

and long-term outcomes. Complex traumatic exposure refers to children's experiences of multiple traumatic events that occur within the caregiving system—the social environment that is supposed to be the source of safety and stability in a child's life. Typically, complex trauma exposure refers to the simultaneous or sequential occurrences of child maltreatment—including emotional abuse and neglect, sexual abuse, physical abuse, and witnessing domestic violence—that are chronic and begin in early childhood.

(2003, p. 13)

These childhood survivors of complex trauma often present with more significant somatic symptoms (e.g., insomnia, agitation, headaches, stomach and back pain, and autoimmune disorders, to name a few), more problems in affect (e.g., depression, hopelessness, anger, self-hatred, alienation, and inability to self-regulate), more dissociation/specific changes in states of consciousness, more cognitive issues (e.g., learning difficulties, "deformations of identity" and "a malignant sense of self, guilt and evil," low self-esteem, and shame), relational complaints (e.g., fear of abandonment and domination, trust, emotional connections to others), and more "unstable relationships" than those suffering from "simple PTSD" (Herman, 1992). As Herman summarizes, "After prolonged and repeated trauma, by contrast, survivors may be at risk for repeated harm, either self-inflicted [such as suicide] or at the hands of others" (p. 388).

In 2002, The National Child Traumatic Stress Network did a survey on "complex trauma exposure, outcomes and treatment approaches" for children receiving assessment and intervention. Their studies disclosed that 78% had been subject to "multiple and/or prolonged trauma" and that 98% of the clinicians servicing this population conclude average onset occurred before the age of 11, while 93% of the clinicians reported average onset before the age of 8. This survey further revealed, according to the National Child Traumatic Stress Network, "that a large percentage of trauma exposed children exhibit several forms of posttraumatic sequelae not captured by standard PTSD, depression or anxiety disorder diagnoses," and that 50% or more of the children surveyed showed notable disturbances in "affect regulation, attention and concentration, negative self-image, impulse control, aggression and risk taking behaviors" (NCTSN, 2012)

In his 2003 article, "The Neurobiology of Childhood Trauma and Abuse," van der Kolk both supports Herman's significant contributions and offers additional potent insight regarding our understanding of the world of childhood trauma. As van der Kolk notes, "Trauma exposure affects what children anticipate and focus on and how they organize the way they appraise and process information. Trauma-induced alterations in threat perceptions are expressed in how they think, feel, behave, and regulate their biological systems" (p. 293). Van der Kolk focuses on "the developmental neurobiology of PTSD" on children such as "the maturation of specific structures at particular ages," their "physiologic and neuroendocrinologic responses," (p. 294) and on their ability to "coordinate cognition, emotion regulation, and behaviors " (p. 294). Van der Kolk also maintains that "biology shapes perception." As van der Kolk explains, "The biological structures that are on-line to interpret the meaning of sensory input determine how children perceive, remember, and integrate new experiences into the totality of the personality" (p. 297). He also addresses how complex trauma in children perpetuates a lack of self-regulation, how their learning and memory processes and social dysfunction are impacted by this trauma, and how this population is more susceptible to physical illness. Moreover, van der Kolk guides us through understanding the role of parts of the brain in a traumatized child such as the brain stem, midbrain, parasympathetic nervous system, the hypothalamic-pituitary-adrenal axis, the limbic system, the hippocampus, the prefrontal cortex, the cerebellum, and the corpus callosum in an effort to help clinicians better understand the biological and somatic implications of trauma, and to help these prolonged traumatized children acquire an "awareness of who they are and what has happened to them, to learn to observe what is happening in present time and physically respond to current demands instead of recreating the traumatic past behaviorally, emotionally and biologically" (van der Kolk, 2003). As van der Kolk concludes, "Much of the impact of trauma is on the subcortical structures and on the degree to which cortical and cerebellar structures can help the growing child modulate his or her limbic, midbrain, and brain stem responses to danger and fear" (p. 309).

As a proponent of *integrated* and systemic thinking, I believe it is essential to keep a keen eye on the family system at all times when considering the discussions of both Herman and van der Kolk (e.g., which family member or members were responsible for the trauma, the parental reaction to the trauma, and the childhood trauma[s] and psychopathology of the parents themselves) as well as to utilize comprehensive assessments and trauma treatments and interventions, when working with complex childhood trauma (Cook et al., 2005).

A study by Sherman et al. (2006), examined the *interpersonal* effects of trauma among members of the armed forces returning from Iraq and Afghanistan. They concluded that domestic violence, hostility (most likely a result of a partner's attempt at reengagement), marital instability, relationship dissatisfaction rates, and negative intimacy issues were much higher (45%) than those found in veterans not suffering from trauma. This may suggest a heightened risk to their family members when it comes to their own development of complex trauma. The presence of secondary traumatic stress suggests that family members in close contact with a traumatized person, who chronically encounter their trauma-induced behaviors, will often experience similar symptoms since they come to identify with the experiences of the victim and begin to internalize them. Note that high levels of secondary trauma are found in one-third of spouses of Holocaust survivors (Goff and Smith, 2005; Lev-Wiesel and Amir, 2001).

In their highly perceptive study, Goff and Smith (2005) developed the Couple Adaptation to Traumatic Stress Model, or CATS. This model helps track variables such as pre-disposing factors (e.g., individual characteristics, unresolved stress experience, and preexisting vulnerabilities) and resources (e.g., financial, educational, social support, and coping strategies), level of functioning (e.g., emotional, behavioral, and cognitive) in both primary and secondary trauma survivors. These variables were deemed to meaningfully impact the interpersonal relationship of the couple, thus measuring the potential for a mutual process of individual trauma symptoms of both partners and supporting a systemic theory of traumatic stress (Goff and Smith, 2005). And, as we have just seen, such secondary trauma can turn out to be an instance of complex trauma if the victim of the primary trauma visits his or her post-traumatic behaviors on family members on a regular basis.

Extricating marital problems or relational difficulties from trauma-related difficulties is a challenge. Research clearly shows that the relational life of clients affected by traumatic experiences often revolves around their subjective experiences of the traumatic events(s). It changes how clients see themselves, how they see the world around themselves and how they interact with those around them. These challenges will be addressed in Chapter 6 when I utilize the Metaframeworks perspective, not yet often utilized by clinicians or researchers to enhance the effectiveness of EMDR in healing trauma in external family systems.

Although psychological trauma and PTSD almost always present with severe comorbid mental health diagnoses, as I mentioned in my Introduction and have found to be the case in my clinical practice, there remains little in the way of research on the relationship of comorbidity to complex or chronic trauma (see Chapter 6). Bessel A. van der Kolk, Susan Roth, David Pelcovitz, Susanne Sunday, and Joseph Spinazzola in their 2005 study, "Disorders of Extreme Distress: The Empirical Foundation of a Complex Adaptation to Trauma," however, acknowledge the issue of comorbidity in PTSD and the need for "further exploration of what constitutes effective treatment of the full spectrum of posttraumatic psychopathology" based on the fact that "children and adults exposed to chronic interpersonal trauma consistently demonstrate psychological disturbances that are not captured in the posttraumatic stress disorder (PTSD) diagnosis" (p. 389). As they continue to explain, "In the PTSD literature, psychiatric problems that do not fall within the framework of PTSD are generally referred to as 'comorbid conditions,' as if they occurred independently from the PTSD symptoms" (p. 390). This suggests the necessity of utilizing trauma treatments that are inclusive, since the National Comorbidity Survey (Kessler et al., 1995) "found that approximately 84% of people with PTSD had another lifetime diagnosis" (p. 1049).

Staggering Statistics

Trauma is ubiquitous even in a relatively stable country such as the United States. The website Addiction Hope reports that

> two-thirds of . . . children experienced at least one traumatic event by age 16, including 30.8% with exposure to one event and 37% to multiple

events. The most common events were witnessing or learning about a trauma that affected others, known as 'vicarious' events. Children who experience trauma are often those with depressive, disruptive behavior disorders and high anxiety. . . . In the United States, approximately five million children experience some form of traumatic event each year.

(Addiction Hope, 2004)

In their 2016 posting, "Suicide: 2016 Facts and Figures," the American Foundation for Suicide Prevention lists suicide as the 10th leading cause of death in the United States (American Foundation for Suicide Prevention, 2016). In his 2008 study, "Epidemiology of the Relationship between Traumatic Experience and Suicidal Behaviors," Kerry L. Knox addresses the risk factors for suicide among those who suffered from childhood trauma, i.e., physical, sexual, and emotional abuse. As Knox recognizes, "up to 80% of the risk for suicide would be eliminated if the abuse during childhood was eliminated" (p. 2). Knox further calls our attention to many studies that establish a relationship between trauma and suicide in those experiencing the "adverse childhood experiences," including a (2008) study conducted by Afifi et al. whose purpose was "to determine the fractions of psychiatric disorders and suicide ideation and attempts in a general population sample attributable to childhood physical abuse, sexual abuse, and witnessing domestic violence" (p. 3). Afifi et al., who obtained their data from the U.S. National Comorbidity Survey Replication, concluded that "having experienced any adverse event [above] accounted for a substantial proportion of suicide ideation and attempts among women (16% and 50%, respectively) and men (21% and 33%, respectively)" (p. 3). Knox also points out that "the literature from military and veteran populations provides evidence that these are important populations in which to consider assessing for suicidal behaviors" (p. 3). Knox's view's in general are supported by the National Center for PTSD which maintains that "the finding pointed to a robust relationship between PTSD and suicide after controlling for comorbid disorders" (Hudenko et al., 2016). Furthermore, their 2016 study "The Relationship between PTSD and Suicide," the National Center for PTSD posits the connection between PTSD and the suicide risk in veterans and calls our attention to studies that explore this connection. The problem remains, however, according to Knox, that "many of these studies on trauma and suicide rely on self-reported data of an attempted suicide. Currently there is no central registry of attempted suicide events in the United States that might serve to validate studies that use suicide attempts as an outcome that may occur years after exposure to trauma" (p. 2).

According to the American Psychological Association, drawing on data from the book *After the Crash: Psychological Assessment and Treatment of Survivors of Motor Vehicle Accidents,* by Edward Blanchard et al., "Motor Vehicle accidents (MVAs) have been found to be the single leading cause of PTSD in the general population." They are the most frequent, directly experienced trauma for men and the second most frequent trauma for women (APA, 2004).

Violence is obviously a potent source of trauma, and it is literally costly: intimate partner violence was estimated to cost $8.3 billion in 2003. That figure includes the costs of mental health services and lost productivity (SAMHSA, 2015). Recent reports on partner violence in the United States suggest that somewhere between 9% and 44% of women are victims of domestic violence, depending on how one chooses to define it (SAMHSA, 2015).

Warfare is the trauma source that most quickly comes to mind for many of us. In a 2004 posting on the Addiction Hope website, "Trauma Causes, Statistics, Signs, Symptoms and Side-effects," it is reported that, "In many countries that have experienced war, more than 60% of the children are displaced and traumatized." In "Veterans Fail to Seek Care for PTSD," a 2008 study conducted by the Rand Corporation and posted on the Psych Central website, it was found that "researchers have determined that nearly 20 percent of military members who have returned from Iraq and Afghanistan report symptoms of post-traumatic stress disorder or major depression, yet only slightly more than half have sought treatment" (p. 1). According to this same study,

> Service members reported exposure to a wide variety of traumatic events while deployed, with half saying they had a friend who was seriously wounded or killed, 45 percent reported they saw dead or seriously injured non-combatants, and over 10 percent saying they were injured themselves and required hospitalization. Rates of PTSD and major depression were highest among Army soldiers and Marines, and among service members who were no longer on active duty (people in the reserves and those who had been discharged or retired from the military).
>
> (p. 2)

In her 2016 account of the latest research on Veterans with PTSD in *New Scientist*, Jessica Hamzelou reports that, on average, an incredible "20 US veterans with PTSD take their own lives each day" (p. 38).

As such, "The RAND report recommends the military create a system that would allow service members to receive mental health services confidentially in order to ease concerns about negative career repercussions" (Psych Central, 2008, p. 2).

Nor should we overlook the significant impact that trauma has upon physical health. It is a culprit in chronic conditions including diabetes and heart disease. At the same time, disease can produce trauma. The World Health organization calculates that approximately 35 million people have died of AIDS (Cook et al., 2016). As a result, countless relatives and friends of the victims have become secondary trauma victims.

Children who grow up with an alcoholic parent are at risk for trauma. The National Institute on Alcohol Abuse and Alcoholism found that in 2012 more than 10% of U.S. children found themselves in this unfortunate position. According to the Center for Behavioral Health Statistics and Quality, that comes to over 7 million children.

The latest scientific research, as reported in a 2016 issue of *New Scientist*, on susceptibility to developing PTSD focuses on a host of factors including gender, childhood experience, genetics, epigenetics, and, even, hormones. As Jessica Hamzelou explains in her article "The Aftermath," "Even in cases of accidents, physical assaults, disaster or fire, women are more prone to PTSD than men." She goes on to observe, however, "But there could be a genetic component too. Several genes have been linked to PTSD, and the condition runs in families. Research in identical twins suggests that about 30 per cent of the variants in risk is down to genetics" (p. 40). Even hormones seem to play a role. "The difference seems," continues Hamzelou, "to be down to oestrogen [British spelling]: the bit of DNA that the hormone can bind to is different in the vulnerable gene variant. . . That may help explain why women with PTSD report feeling more anxious when they have low levels of the hormone, such as before a period" (p. 40). But there is more, "As well as genetics and hormones," continues Hamzelou,

> epigenetics—the study of how our environment and experiences can modify the way our genes work—could hold clues to why some people have a higher risk of PTSD. Childhood abuse seems to prime adults in this way. In a study of people who developed PTSD after several traumatic experiences as adults, those who were abused in childhood had more epigenetic changes related to immune regulation and central nervous system development. They also had more changes overall: 12 times as many as those who faced trauma only as adults.
>
> (p. 41)

Hamzelou further notes that "PTSD can also modify the expression of genes involved in cognition and immune function, which may underlie symptoms such as difficulty concentrating and poor health" (p. 41).

While figures for violence and trauma have already been provided, we end our survey of trauma statistics with what might well be considered the emblematic form of traumatic experience in the United States today, namely, mass shootings. On July 18, 1984, 21 persons were killed and 19 wounded by a shooter at a McDonald's restaurant in San Ysidro, California. Edmond, Oklahoma, saw gun violence on August 20, 1986 that left 14 dead and 6 wounded. Ten people were killed and 4 wounded in Jacksonville, Florida on June 18, 1990. On October 16, 1991, 22 people were killed and 20 wounded in Killeen, Texas. November 1, 1991, saw 4 killed and 2 injured in Iowa City, Iowa. May 1, 1992, brought gun violence to Olivehurst, California, where 4 were killed and 10 wounded. Eight people were killed and another 6 injured in San Francisco on July 1,1993. There were 6 killed and 19 injured in a gun attack in Garden City, New York, on December 7, 1993. Two middle school students killed 5 and injured 10 in a gun assault in Jonesboro, Arkansas, on March 24, 1998. One of the most notorious shooting incidents in U.S. history took place on April 20, 1999, when two high school students opened fire at their school in Columbine, Colorado, killing 13 people and injuring another 24. July 29, 1999, saw 9 killed and 12 injured in an attack in Atlanta, and September 15 of the same year brought death to 7, with another 7 injured, in a gun attack in Fort Worth, Texas. Yet again in 1999, this time on November 2 in Honolulu, a gunman killed 7. On December 26, 2000, an attacker shot and killed 7 co-workers in Wakefield, Massachusetts. 2001 saw 2 killed and 13 injured in Santee, California, while 3 were shot to death in Tucson on October 28, 2002. In 2003, 5 were killed and 9 injured in Meridian, Mississippi. Nine people were shot to death and 7 injured on the Red Lake Indian Reservation in Minnesota on March 21, 2005. Goleta, California, witnessed the death of 6 people on January 30, 2006. Five people were killed and 5 more injured in Nickel Mines, Pennsylvania, on October 2, 2006, and another 5 were killed and 4 injured in Salt Lake City on February 12, 2007. In a widely covered college shooting on April 16, 2007, 32 were killed and 17 injured in Blacksburg, Virginia. A gunman killed 8 and wounded 4 in an Omaha shopping mall filled with holiday shoppers on December 5, 2007. Another college shooting, this time on February 14, 2008, in DeKalb, Illinois, left 5 dead and 16 injured. On April 3, 2009, 13 were killed and 4 injured at an immigration center in Binghamton, New York. Thirteen were killed and 32 injured in a Ft. Hood, Texas shooting on November 5, 2009. Three were killed and 3 wounded in Huntsville, Alabama on February 12, 2010, with another 8 killed and 2 injured in Manchester, Connecticut, on August 3 of the same year. 2011 brought 6 killed and 11 injured in Tucson on January 8, and 8 were killed and 1 injured in Seal Beach, California. 2012 proved no better, with 7 killed and 3 injured in Oakland on April 2, and 12 killed and 58 injured on July 20 in Aurora, Colorado. Still in 2012, 6 were killed and 3 injured on August 5 in Oak Creek, Wisconsin, with another 6 killed and 2 injured on September 28 in Minneapolis, and 3 killed and 4 injured on October 21 in Brookfield, Wisconsin. Then on December 14, 2012, a lone gunman killed 26 and injured 1 at the Sandy Hook Elementary School in Newtown, Connecticut. Twenty of those killed were first graders (see Appendix 1). The year 2013 brought 5 dead in a gun incident on June 7 in Santa Monica, and 13 dead and 3 injured in Washington, D.C. on September 16. On April 2, 2014, gun violence returned to Ft. Hood, Texas, with 3 killed and 16 injured. Later in the same year, on May 23, 6 were killed and 7 wounded in Isla Vista, California. June 18, 2015 saw 9 killed in Charlestown, South Carolina. And on July 16 of the same year 5 were shot to death and 3 injured in Chattanooga, Tennessee. Again, this time on October 1, 9 were killed and 9 injured in Roseburg, Oregon. December 2, 2015, brought the San Bernadino shooting spree that killed 14 people and wounded 22 more. On June 12, 2016, the worst mass shooting in modern U.S. history occurred when a gunman killed 50 and injured 53 at a nightclub in Orlando, Florida. On September 30, 2016, a South Carolina teen killed his father before shooting 6-year-old Jacob Hall, at Townville Elementary School. Jacob later died from the bullet which hit his femoral artery. Since then, over 20 other such shootings have occurred, culminating in the worst mass shooting in modern U.S. history in Las Vegas on October 1, 2017. (Each of these incidents are widely referenced on the internet).

References

Addiction Hope. (2004). "Trauma Causes, Statistics, Signs, Symptoms and Side-Effects." www.addictionhope.com/trauma/ Accessed on September 6, 2016.

American Foundation for Suicide Prevention. (2016). "Suicide: 2016 Facts and Figures." https://afsp.org/wp-content/uploads/2016 Accessed June 12 2017.

American Psychological Association. (2004). "After the Crash: Psychological Assessment and Treatments of Survivors of Motor Vehicle Accidents." www.apa.org Accessed on September 6, 2016.

"Complex Trauma in Children and Adolescents: White Paper from the National Child Traumatic Stress Network Complex Trauma Task Force." (2003). *The National Child Traumatic Stress Network*, 4–40.

Cook, A., Spinazzola, J., Ford, J., Lanktree, C., Blaustein, M., Cloitre, M., et al. (2005). "Complex Trauma in Children and Adolescents," *Psychiatric Annals, 35* (5), 390–398.

Cook, A., Spinazzola, J., Ford, J., Lanktree, C., Blaustein, M., Cloitre, M., DeRosa, R., Hubbard, R., & Global Health Observatory (GHO) Data: HIV/AIDS. (2016). *World Health Organization*. www.who.int/gho/hiv/en/ Accessed on December 23, 2015.

Goff, B.S., & Smith, D.B. (2005). "Systemic Traumatic Stress: The Couple Adaptation to Traumatic Stress Model." *Journal of Marital and Family Therapy, 31*, 145–157.

Hamzelou, J. (2016). "Why Women Are More at Risk of PTSD—and How to Prevent It." *New Scientist*, September 14, 38–40.

Hanson, T.C., Hessebrook, M., Tworkowsi, & Swan, S. (2002). "The Prevalence and Management of Trauma, in the Public Domain: An Agency and Clinical Perspective." *Journal of Behavioral Health Services and Research, 29*, 365–380.

Herman, J.L. (1992). "Complex PTSD: A Syndrome in Survivors of Prolonged and Repeated Trauma." *Journal of Traumatic Stress, 5* (3), 377–391.

Herman, J.L., Perry, J.C., & van der Kolk, B.A. (1989). "Childhood Trauma in Borderline Personality Disorder." *American Journal of Psychiatry, 146* (4), 490–495.

Hudenko, H., Homaifar, B., & Wortzel, H. (2016). "The Relationship between PTSD and Suicide." *National Center for PTSD*. www.ptsd.va.gov/professional/co-occuring/ptsd-suicide.asp Accessed on March 9, 2017.

Kessler, R.C., Sonnega, A., Bromet, E., Hughes, M., & Nelson, C.B. (1995). "Posttraumatic Stress Disorder in the National Comorbidity Survey." *Archives of General Psychiatry, 52*, 1048–1060.

Knox, K.L. (2008). "Epidemiology of the Relationship between Traumatic Experience and Suicidal Behaviors." *PTSD Research Quarterly, 19* (4), 1–8.

Levine, P.A. (2010). *In an Unspoken Voice: How the Body Releases Trauma and Restores Goodness*. Berkeley, CA: North Atlantic Books.

Levine, P.A. (2015). *Trauma and Memory: Brain and Body in a Search for a Living Past*. Berkeley, CA: North Atlantic Books.

Lev-Wiesel, R., & Amir, M. (2001). "Secondary Traumatic Stress, Psychological Distress, Sharing of Traumatic Reminisces and Marital Quality among Spouses of Holocaust Child Survivors." *Journal of Marital and Family Therapy, 27*, 433–444.

Psych Central. (2008). "Veterans Fail to Seek Care for PTSD." www.psychcentral.com/news/2008/04/18/veterans-fail-to-seek-care-forptsd/2166.html Accessed on September 6, 2016.

Sherman, M.D., Sautter, F., Jackson, M.H., Lyons, J., & Hans, X. (2006). "Domestic Violence in Veterans with PTSD Who Seek Couple Therapy." *Journal of Marital and Family Therapy*, 32, 5–16.

Substance Abuse and Mental Health Services Administration (SAMHSA). (2015). "Trauma and Violence." www.samhsa.gov/trauma-violence Accessed on September 6, 2016.

"Suicide: 2016 Facts and Figures." *American Foundation for Suicide Prevention.* www.afsp.org/wp-content/uploads/2016/06/2016-National-facts-Figures.pdf Accessed on March 9, 2017.

van der Kolk, B.A. (2003). "The Neurobiology of Childhood Trauma and Abuse." *Child and Adolescent Psychiatric Clinics of North America*, 12, 293–317.

van der Kolk, B.A., Roth, S., Pelcovitz, D., Sunday, S., & Spinazzola, J. (2005). "Disorders of Extreme Stress: The Empirical Foundation of a Complex Adaptation to Trauma." *Journal of Traumatic Stress*, 18 (5), 389–399.

Wilson, J.P., & Keane, T.M. (2004). *Assessing Psychological Trauma and PTSD.* New York: Guilford Press.

Government and Organizational Resources

American Psychological Association (2008) (2018).
California Evidence-based Clearinghouse for Child Welfare (2010).
CCrest (2003).
Center for Behavioral Health Statistics and Quality (2012).
Centers for Disease Control and Prevention (2014).
Department of Health and Human Services (HHS) (2012).
Department of Veterans Affairs and Department of Defense (2010).
National Center for PTSD (2015).
The National Child Traumatic Stress Network (NCTSN) (2012).
National Criminal Justice Reference Service (2011).
National Institute of Mental Health NIMH (2015).
National Institute on Alcohol Abuse and Alcoholism (NIH) (2012).
SAMHSA's National Registry of Evidence-based Programs and Practices (2011).
United Kingdom Department of Health (2010).
World Health Organization (WHO) (2013).

2 Quagmires in Attempting to Heal the Traumatized Brain

DSM-V

Classification systems, as such, often present complexity and raise ethical and diagnostic questions. Developing a classification system for mental health disorders such as the DSM-V is no exception. The first attempt to create a classification of mental disorders took the form of collecting statistics in 1840, and resulted in a census that identified a single diagnosis, "idiocy/insanity." This attempt was followed by an 1880 census which put forth the existence of seven mental health disorders in the U.S. population. These disorders included mania, melancholia, monomania, paresis, dementia, dipsomania, and epilepsy (from American Psychiatric Association as reported in *Wikipedia*, 2016).

The Diagnostic and Statistical Manual of Mental Disorders (DSM-I), published by the American Psychiatric Committee on Nomenclature and Statistics, was not available until 1952. Its subsequent versions DSM-II (1968), DSM-III (1980), DSM-III-R (1987), DSM-IV (1994), DSM-IV-TR (2000) followed. These versions of the DSM were coordinated around another mental health diagnostic manual, the *International Classification of Diseases* (ICD-6) (Wikipedia, 2016).

The DSM has morphed over the years into its current and fifth iteration, the DSM-V that includes 20 chapters, which was published on May 18, 2013. The DSM-V was the culmination of data from 400 research investigators, namely psychiatrists and other mental health professionals and 13 conferences supported by the National Institute of Health (NIH). The DSM-V was monitored by a 2007 APA-formed 27-member Task Force whose focus was on mental health disorders apparently related to one another as reflected by similarities related to vulnerabilities and symptom characteristics. The DSM-V more closely aligns with the World Health Organization's (WHO) eleventh edition of the ICD-II in an attempt to recognize the scientific origins of diseases and their pathologies. The intent of this alignment was to eliminate the complication of replicating scientific results with two separate manuals. The DSM-V locates new areas of study, qualifies new disorders as well as removing others, addresses more cultural and gender-specific meaning-making, rearranges the order of the chapters in an effort to better address disorders' relatedness to one another, and coordinates with the ICD-II in order to achieve better communication and use of diagnoses across disorders, and removes the multiaxial system of the DSM-IV-TR, to name but a few changes.

The DSM-V is clearly intended as a guidebook for mental health professionals, researchers, psychiatric drug regulation agencies, health insurance companies, and the legal system to classify and diagnose mental health disorders. It remains, however, a manual that raises complex diagnostic, content-related, and ethical questions and, as such, is surrounded by much controversy. According to Christopher Lane, writing for *Psychology Today* in 2013, for instance, there are ongoing issues about the DSM-V such as the reliability and the validity of its diagnostic categories, its over-dependence on symptomology, its cultural bias, and the fact that the National Institute of Mental Health (NIMH) withdrew its support for the DSM-V just two weeks before its publication (Lane, 2013).

As Erin Anderssen also pre-emptively states in "Five Things You Should Know About the New DSM Mental-Health Bible," "Critics have decried the final draft as 'hopelessly flawed' warning it [DSM-V] may lead to unnecessary treatments" (Anderssen, 2012, p. 1). Critics, including the National Institute of Mental Health (NIMH), argue the DSM-V represents an "unscientific and subjective system." Many other critics feel, as do I, that these changes also suggest that clients are being over-diagnosed, pathologized, made dependent on the pharmaceutical industry, and are being challenged by insurers such as Medicare and Medicaid as to whether they will be reimbursed for their treatments.

In a 2014 interview with David Bullard, "Bessel van der Kolk on Trauma, Development and Healing," posted on *psychotherapy.net*, van der Kolk recounts the narrative of his efforts in 2009 to have "Developmental Trauma Disorder" added to the DSM-V and after having "marshaled a lot of support, such as that from the National Association of State Mental Health Program Directors, who serve 6.1 million people annually, with a combined budget of $29.5 billion," the APA turned him down.

In addition, in their 2005 article "Disorders of Extreme Stress: The Empirical Foundation of a Complex Adaptation to Trauma," Bessel A. van der Kolk, Susan Roth, David Pelcovitz, Susanne Sunday, and Joseph Spinazzola report that "children and adults exposed to chronic interpersonal trauma consistently demonstrate disturbances that [were] not captured in the post-traumatic stress disorder (PTSD) diagnosis" (p. 389). This is difficult to digest given that the American Psychiatric Association (APA) conducted, as van der Kolk et al., 2005 point out, a field trial in 1994 for PTSD studying these disturbances and demonstrating other meaning-making connections when they selected

> 400 treatment-seeking traumatized individuals and 128 community residents and found that victims of prolonged interpersonal trauma, particularly trauma early in the life cycle, had a high incidence of problems

with (a) regulation of affect and impulses, (b) memory and attention, (c) self-perception, (d) interpersonal relations, (e) somatization, and (f) systems of meaning. This raises important issues about the categorical versus the dimensional nature of posttraumatic stress, as well as the issue of comorbidity in PTSD. These data invite further exploration of what constitutes effective treatment of the full spectrum of posttraumatic psychopathology.

(p. 389)

This DSM-IV Field Trial, conducted between 1990 and 1992, demonstrated that prolonged trauma and the number of traumas experienced at an early onset, before the age of 14, impacted psychological functioning such as affect regulation, dissociation, and somatization quite apart from PTSD symptomology. The DSM-V, however, still puts forth limited assessment/diagnosis and attention regarding traumatized children and even less around their having co-morbidity with other mental health disorders such as depression, anxiety, substance abuse, panic attacks, eating and dissociative disorder, and potential for latent bipolar and personality disorders. As any clinician knows, many disorders present simultaneously. Given this, it is hard to imagine not addressing the comorbidity factor as it relates to PTSD. Yet, there is little reliable and valid research in PTSD literature which discusses problems such as "disturbances in perception, information processing, affect regulation, impulse control, and personality development" (as measured in the study) as well as the comorbidity factor with PTSD. By not continuing the path of those conducting the aforementioned field trial studies such as the one briefly summarized, we actually prevent clinicians from having a successful treatment approach in healing not only this population, but all those who suffer from psychological trauma (van der Kolk et al., 2005).

There is one contribution in the DSM-V, however, that does matter given the premise of this book and especially as it relates to the utilization and efficacy of EMDR. That contribution relates to the "many changes to PTSD criteria." According to Ashley A. Houston, Jennifer Webb-Murphey, and Eileen Delaney in their 2015 resource article "From DSM-IV-TR to DSM-V: Changes in Posttraumatic Stress Disorder," written for the Naval Center for Combat & Operational Stress Control (NCCOSC), "revisions include changes to the language in Criterion A, in which a traumatic event is now more clearly defined than it was in the DSM-IV-TR. The DSM-V specifies examples of experiencing or witnessing a traumatic event, such as sexual assault or repeated indirect exposure to adverse events such as in the case for professionals (e.g., first responders), and requires being explicit about how the event was experienced (i.e., directly or indirectly)" (Houston et al., 2015). The most important changes made in the DSM-V regarding the diagnosis of PTSD, recognized by these authors as well as the author of this book, are the addition of another cluster, the reframing of others, and the addition of subtypes of PTSD such as the pre-school subtype in children younger than six and the dissociative subtype. As Houston et al. note, for example, "*Intrusive symptoms* (formerly 're-experiencing') and *alterations in arousal and reactivity* (formerly 'arousal') remain as clusters, while *avoidance and numbing* have been split into two clusters, *avoidance* (Criterion C) and *negative alterations in cognitions and mood* (Criterion D)." Evidence-based treatments for PTSD, such as EMDR and the integration of EMDR with cognitive behavioral therapy, rely on the recognition of these cognitions in therapy. Furthermore, the new symptoms included in Criterion D, "distorted blame of self or others for causing the traumatic event or for resulting consequences, and persistent (and often distorted) negative beliefs and expectations about oneself or the world" (Houston, et al. 2015) play a crucial and integral part in the EMDR protocol that I will focus on in the next chapter on EMDR.

Despite these efforts to introduce new criteria in the diagnosis of PTSD, however, trauma remains inadequately accounted for in the DSM-V. As van der Kolk notes in *The Body Keeps the Score: Brain, Mind and the Body in the Healing of Trauma* (2014):

> Even before DSM-V was released, the *American Journal of Psychiatry* published the results of validity tests of various new diagnoses, which indicated that the DSM-V largely lacks what in the world of science is known as "reliability"—the ability to produce consistent, replicable results. In other words, it lacks scientific validity.
>
> (pp. 164–165)

As van der Kolk further points out, "If you pay attention only to faulty biology and defective genes as the cause of mental problems and ignore abandonment, abuse and deprivation, you are likely to run into as many dead ends as previous generations did blaming it on terrible mothers" (p. 165). This oversight in the DSM-V leaves trauma further under-diagnosed, thus accounting for the fact that it is largely ignored in treatment plans, as I pointed out in Chapter 1. As a result, people remain stuck in their trauma and stagnant in their lives, although we know that memory research suggests that all memories are fluid and can be changed, a matter also addressed in Chapter 1.

In his book *In an Unspoken Voice: How the Body Releases Trauma and Restores Goodness (2010)*, Peter A. Levine captures another crucial missing piece from the DSM-V's diagnosis of trauma. As Levine notes,

> The previous versions of the PTSD diagnosis have been careful not to suggest a mechanism (or even a theory) to explain what happens in the brain and body when people become traumatized. This absence is important for more than academic reasons: a theory suggests rationales for treatment and prevention. This avoidance and sole reliance on taxonomy is an understandable overreaction to the Freudian theory's previous stranglehold on psychology.
>
> (p. 29)

According to Levine, "Most people think of trauma as a 'mental' problem, even as a 'brain disorder.' However, trauma is something that also happens in the body. We become stiff or, alternately, we collapse, overwhelmed and defeated with helpless dread. Either way, trauma defeats life" (p. 31). As Levine passionately puts it, "To these people, who live in a cage of anxiety, fear, pain and shame, I hope to convey a deeper appreciation that their lives are not dominated by a 'disorder' but by *an injury that can be transformed and healed!*" (p. 12; see Chapters 1, 3, and 4).

Why Talk Therapy Alone Does Not Work

A traumatic experience leaves so much more than a mere bad memory of a past event. Trauma affects the person far beyond the cognitive level, wreaking havoc on the mind, brain, and body as a whole. In her 2008 internet posting, "How Trauma Impacts the Brain" (talking points from a seminar for Rachel's Vineyard Ministries), Theresa Burke offers this synthesis:

> Trauma disrupts the stress-hormone system. It plays havoc with the entire nervous system, which prevents people from processing and integrating traumatic memories into conscious mental frameworks. Traumatic memories stay "stuck" in the brain's nether regions—the nonverbal, nonconscious, subcortical regions (amygdala, thalamus, hippocampus, hypothalamus and brain stem)—where they are not accessible to the frontal lobes—the understanding, thinking, reasoning parts of the brain.
>
> (p. 1)

Thus traumas are just as much physiological in nature as they are psychological, causing a shift of the body's norm to one of hyper-arousal, disorganization, and disintegration. Solely using talk therapy to treat a traumatized person is like trying to teach someone with a broken leg how to run; as hard as you try to teach and help that person, your efforts will be futile until their broken leg has healed. Talk therapy will be unsuccessful in reaching a person's physiological and psychological wounds until the physiological wounds have first been mended.

Burke's ideas are underscored and supported by van der Kolk when he informs us: "fundamentally, words can't integrate the disorganized sensations and action patterns that form the imprint of trauma" (as quoted in Wylie, 2015, p. 6). As van der Kolk continues, "The imprint of trauma doesn't 'sit' in the verbal, understanding, part of the brain, but in the much deeper regions—amygdala, hippocampus, hypothalamus, brain stem which are only marginally affected by thinking and cognition" (as quoted in Wylie, 2015, p. 8). Thus, talk therapy alone cannot treat the trauma because "it doesn't go deep enough into the survival brain. Treatment needs to integrate the sensations and actions that have become stuck, so that people can regain a sense of familiarity and efficacy in their 'organism'" (as quoted in Wylie, 2015, p. 8).

In 2015, the senior editor of the *Psychotherapy Networker*, Mary Sykes Wylie, recounted van der Kolk's story of working with veterans and "the treatment that he felt was not really helping his patients to move on." "It was standard talk therapy 101," continues Wylie,

> helping them explore their thoughts and feelings—supplemented with group therapy and medications. During individual sessions with clients, he often focused intensely on patients' past traumas, in the interest of getting them to process and integrate their memories, realizing that many of these patients got worse and suicide attempts increased.
>
> (as quoted by Wylie, p. 8)

In a 2014 interview with David Bullard posted on *psychotherapy.net*, van der Kolk notes, "Of course, talking can be very helpful in acknowledging the reality about what's happened and how it's affected you, but talking about it doesn't put it behind you." Furthermore, as van der Kolk continues,

> Cognitive Behavioral Therapy (and "Trauma Focused CBT") talk therapies, and prolonged exposure therapies can make some changes in people's distress, but traumatic stress has little to do with cognition—it emanates from the emotional part of the brain that is rewired to constantly send out messages of dangers and distress, with the result that it becomes difficult to feel fully alive in the present. Blasting people with the memories of the trauma may lead to desensitization and numbing, but it does not lead to integration: an organic awareness that the event is over, and that you are fully alive in the present.
>
> (van der Kolk, 2014)

Another population that I have discovered in my clinical practice that can actually get worse with talk therapy alone is those with Borderline Personality Disorder. While they are feared among many clinicians because of their erratic and impossibly resistant behaviors in the clinical setting, they are actually quite helpless and are suffering from something much deeper. Most of them, for instance, are, in fact, suffering from extreme physical, sexual, and emotional abuse from childhood and in their adult lives, which, as we all know, translates into complex trauma and Posttraumatic Stress Disorder. They often have challenges connecting with others and feeling pleasure, and they present as being distraught and frustrated. Thus, talk therapy alone cannot reverse the devastating changes that wreak havoc on their minds and their physical, emotional, and somatic parts.

According to the discussions regarding the inefficacy of talk therapy to heal those populations suffering from traumatic experiences, for those who often feel helpless, hopeless, unconnected with others, and unable to be happy and in charge of their 'selves,' a neurobiological protocol such as EMDR would seem to offer a world of healing. As Francine Shapiro points out in a 2012 *New York Times* Blog "Expert Answers on EMDR," comparing CBT and EMDR, "EMDR therapy had superior outcomes on at least some measures and/or was more efficient, using fewer sessions in five of the seven studies." Given the findings in this chapter, the next chapter will focus on EMDR, the centerpiece of neurological-based protocols that prove to heal trauma in family systems as well as other therapies, some successful and other not, with an eye on the fact that talk therapy alone does not work.

Medication Isn't Healing Pervasive Trauma

Psychiatry has used medications to treat traumatized people for decades. The problem is that psychiatric medication can only rarely be considered an actual treatment. In most cases, medications are like anesthetics: they may numb the pain but they don't heal the wound. A traumatized person may think that a medication has helped them to feel better, but the improvement is only temporary. Once it wears off, the symptoms return. There is a time and place for medication, and psychiatry has done an astounding job of enabling many with mental health issues to live a life they never would have been able to otherwise. For the treatment of trauma, however, medication is insufficient to address the underlying issues. Clearly, there are artful physicians who succeed in combining what medications have to offer with other essential strategies. An impressive case in point is the work of Frank Guastella Anderson (see Anderson, 2013).

As with any quagmire, controversy abounds. According to Matt Jeffreys, writing for the National Center for PTSD in 2016, "Medications can be used to ameliorate the biological basis for PTSD symptoms along with co-occurring psychiatric diagnoses, and indirectly may benefit psychological and social symptoms as well." He thoughtfully consider variables such as co-morbidity with other mental health diagnoses, the resiliency of individuals with personality disorders, patients' age, symptomology, DSM-V symptom clusters targeted, and the determination of medications. Based on these factors the National Center for PTSD recommends SSRIs like Zoloft, Prozac, and Paxil, approved by the FDA, in order to modulate mood, promote resiliency, and balance serotonergic and noradrenergic transmitters in the nervous system.

The evidence for the effectiveness for Prozac in combat veterans is decidedly mixed. As van der Kolk states, for example, in *The Body Keeps the Score: Brain, Mind and Body in the Healing of Trauma*, "It's interesting that the SSRIs are widely used to treat depression, but in a study in which we compared Prozac with eye movement desensitization and reprocessing (EMDR) for patients with PTSD, many of whom were also depressed, EMDR proved to be a more effective antidepressant than Prozac" (p. 225).

A 2004 article "SSRIs for PTSD: Just How Effective Are They?" posted on *PsychCentral* brings to our attention that only two medications, Zoloft (sertraline) and Paxil (paroxetine), were approved by the FDA for the treatment of trauma. The *PsychCentral* analysis concludes that the evidence for the efficacy of both Zoloft and Paxil in treating PTSD is minimal.

In his 2016 internet post "FDA Warns that Paxil Makes Depressed Adults Suicidal," Peter Breggin takes on the inefficacy of Paxil to a new level when he states,

> In a May 2006 release in collaboration with the manufacturer GlaxoSmith-Kline (GSK), the FDA has acknowledged the antidepressant Paxil causes a statistically significant increased rate of suicidality in depressed adults as measured in controlled clinical trials.
>
> (Breggin, 2006)

Breggin continues to horrify us by revealing that the FDA and GSK continue to obfuscate the true risk in their May 2006 announcement concerning Paxil-induced suicidality in depressed adults. They emphasize the supposedly light increase in suicidality among *young* adults (through age thirty) who take Paxil for a variety of conditions, including for depression, panic attacks, anxiety, and obsessive-compulsive disorder. Far more important is the statistically significant increase in suicidality in all ages of depressed adults. It's worth restating that depressed people getting Paxil are 6.4 times more likely to display suicidal thoughts and behavior than depressed people taking a sugar pill (Breggin, 2006).

In his 2016 internet article "Antidepressants on Trial: Are They a Wonder or a Danger?" appearing on the *New Scientist* site, Robert Whitaker calls our attention to a study conducted more than 10 years ago by the US's National Institute of Mental Health that revealed that "only 26 per cent of patients even responded to an antidepressant, and at the end of the year, only 6 per cent were well." Whitaker also calls attention to the narrative of documentary filmmaker Katinka Blackford Newmann who took the antidepressant Lexapro and "became severely anxious and restless, which are the symptoms of akathisia, a side effect associated with violence and suicide" (Whitaker, 2016).

In the face of such statistics, the National Center for PTSD still considers the use of Remeron and Effexor for co-morbidity with PTSD; mood stabilizers such as Tegretol, Depakote, Lamictal, and Topimax; and benzodiazepines such as Ativan, Klonopin, Xanax, and Valium for anxiety associated with PTSD. They also make the claim that another medication, Prazosin (Minipress), typically given for high blood pressure, can be helpful for specific PTSD symptoms such as nightmares (see Jeffreys, 2016). While PTSD can lead to an increase in adrenaline, which can make you have too many nightmares, in his 2014 article "Prazosin for PTSD" on *WebMD*, Adam Husney agrees that Prazosin may help reduce nightmares but reports: "Prazosin may help your nightmares, but it is not a cure for PTSD and nightmares and anxiety may come back if you stop taking the medication" (Husney, 2014).

Recent research on memory suggests that our memories are not inert units easily accessed, but that they must actually be reassembled each time that we call them up. This has led neuroscientists to begin experiments using another blood pressure medication—propranolol—for "reconsolidation" therapy. The goal is to erase traumatic memories by interfering with the brain's remembering process. Of course, one can ask whether *reprocessing* traumatic memories as accomplished by EMDR is a better avenue to psychological wholeness than simply *wiping out* memories. There are ethical issues as well: should we, for example, erase memories of an act about which we rightly feel guilty, such as a war crime (Phillips, 2017)?

Just how devastating the effects of PTSD can be and how far researchers are willing to go in searching for an effective drug to treat it is evident in a 2016 decision by the U.S. Food and Drug Administration. The agency gave its approval for Phase 3 trials with PTSD sufferers of the drug MDMA, a presently illegal substance better known as Ecstasy, or the "party drug" (Philipps, 2016). Phase 3 testing is the last stage of human research that the FDA requires before considering approving the use of a drug for prescription purposes. Where Ecstasy or MDMA is concerned, this affords the opportunity for large-scale testing and the possibility of statistically significant results. One small study already conducted has been interpreted as suggesting that three carefully supervised doses of Ecstasy can reduce the symptoms of PTSD by over 50% (Philipps, 2016).

In the clinical plan that he proposed for studying the treatment of PTSD with MDMA, Rick Doblin explains that "psychedelic drugs, though each with a unique set of actions and side effects, all serve the generally similar function of increasing access to psychological, emotional processes" (Doblin, 2002). He believes that MDMA may alleviate the fear that human beings feel in response to a perceived threat as it has apparently done with terminal cancer patients (Doblin, 2002).

While, as of this writing, the jury is still out on the effectiveness of Ecstasy as a PTSD treatment, skeptical observers are quick to point out that, because long-term use of the drug has resulted in permanent brain damage in some users, the greatest of caution is necessary in considering Ecstasy for prescription drug status. The unhappy surprises that prescription drugs such as SSRIs have held in store for the medical community, surprises revealed several years after their FDA approval, should only heighten this sense of caution.

In the end, in a 2010 *NPR Fresh Air* Interview, "Psychiatrist Daniel Carlat—A Psychiatrist's Prescription for his Profession," Carlat summarizes the quagmires presented in this chapter in a surprising manner. The interview brings to light several important factors and statistics including that "only 11.5% of all psychiatrists now offer therapy to their patients," and that "we are in the business of making diagnosis using the DSM. . . . And then we usually prescribe medications." As Carlat elaborates,

> We have a conversation (15 or 20) minutes and I ask my patients questions about how they're feeling, what they're thinking, how they're sleeping,

what their concentration level is, what their energy level is, and I pull all those pieces of information together and then I come up with a diagnosis based on the DSM guidebook that we have. And once they have a diagnosis, I match those symptoms up with a medication. So modern psychiatry is really a conversation, a series of symptoms and then a matching process of medication to these symptoms.

(NPR, 2010)

Given the quagmires presented in this chapter, my next chapter will take my readers to a more thoroughly tested and much more effective and *integrated* neurobiological and psychotherapeutic treatment for trauma, EMDR.

References

American Psychiatric Association. (2013). *Diagnostic and Statistical Manual of Mental Disorders (DSM-IV-TR)*. Arlington, VA: APA.

American Psychiatric Association. (2016). *Diagnostic and Statistical Manual of Mental Disorders (DSM-V)*. Arlington, VA: APA.

Anderson, F.H. (2013). "'Who's Taking What?' Connecting Neuroscience, Psychopharmacology and Internal Family Systems for Trauma." Edited by E.L. Ziskind & M. Sweezy. *Internal Family Systems: New Dimensions* (pp. 107–126). New York: Routledge: Taylor & Francis Group.

Anderssen, E. (2012). "Five Things You Should Know about the New DSM Mental Health Bible." *The Globe and Mail*. www.theglobeandmail.com/life/health-and-fitness-health-5-things-you-should-know-about-the-new-dsm-mental-health-bible Accessed on October 5, 2016.

Breggin, P.R. (2006). "FDA Warns That Paxil Makes Depressed Adults Suicidal." www.breggin.com/index.php?option=com_content&task=view&id=60 Accessed on August 25, 2016.

Bullard, D. (2014). "Bessel van der Kolk on Trauma, Development and Healing." www.psychotherapy.net/interview/bessel-van-der-kolk-trauma Accessed on October 5, 2016.

Burke, T. (2008). "How Trauma Impacts the Brain Talking Points from Seminar for Rachel's Vineyard Ministries." www.rachelsvineyard.org/Downloads/CanadaConference08/TextOfBrainPP.pdf Accessed on October 5, 2016.

Doblin, R. (2002). "A Clinical Plan for MDMA (Ecstasy) in the Treatment of Post-Traumatic Stress Disorder (PTSD): Partnering with the FDA." www.maps.org/news-letters/v12n3/12305dob.html Accessed on January 2, 2017.

Houston, M.A., Webb-Murphey, J., & Delany, E. (2015). "From DSM-IV-TR to DSM-5: Changes in Posttraumatic Stress Disorder." *Naval Center for Combat and Operational Stress Control (NCCOSC)*. www.med.navy.mil/sites/nmcd/nccosc/healthprofessionanlsv2/reports/documents/white-paper-from-dsm-iv-tr-to-dsm-v Accessed on October 5, 2016.

Husney, A. (2014). "Prazosin for PTSD." *WebMD*. www.webmd.com/a-z-guides/prazosin/for-ptsd Accessed on October 5, 2016.

Jeffreys, M. (2016). "Clinicians Guide to Medications for PTSD." www.ptsd.va.gov/professional/treatment/overview/clinicians-guide-to-medications-for-psd.asp Accessed on October 5, 2016.

Lane, C. (2013). "The NIMH Withdraws Support for DSM-V." www.psychology-today.com/blog/side-effects/201305/the-nimh/withdraws-support-dsm-v Accessed on February 18, 2017.

Levine, P.A. (2010). *In an Unspoken Voice: How the Body Releases Trauma and Restores Goodness.* Berkeley, CA: North Atlantic Books.

NPR Fresh Air Interview: Psychiatrist Daniel Carlat. (2010). "A Psychiatrists Prescription for His Profession." www.npr.org/templates/story/story.php?storyId=128107547 Accessed on January 5, 2017.

Philipps, D. (2016). "F.D.A. Agrees to New Trials for Ecstasy as Relief for PTSD Patients." www.nytimes.com/2016/11/29/us/ptsd-mdma-ecstasy.html?_r=0 Accessed on November 29, 2016.

Phillips, H. (2017). "Mental Blocks." *New Scientist, 233* (3111), 36–39.

PsychCentral. (2004). "SSRIs for PTSD: Just How Effective Are They?" http://pro.psychcentral.com/ssris-for-PTSD-just-how-effective-are-they/001968.html# Accessed on January 5, 2017.

Shapiro, F. (2012). "Expert Answers on E.M.D.R." *New York Times.* http://consults.blogs.nytimes.com/2012/03/16/expert-answers-on-e-m-d-r/ Accessed on January 4, 2017.

van der Kolk, B.A. (2014). *The Body Keeps the Score: Brain, Mind, and Body in the Healing of Trauma.* New York: Viking.

van der Kolk, B.A., Roth, S., Pelcovitz, D., Sunday, S., & Spinazzola, J. (2005). "Disorders of Extreme Stress: The Empirical Foundation of a Complex Adaptation to Trauma." *Journal of Traumatic Stress, 18* (5), 389–399.

Whitaker, R. (2016). "Antidepressants on Trial: Are They a Wonder or a Danger?" www.newscientist.com/article/mg23130810-600-drug-stories-who-should-we-listen-to/ Accessed on October 5, 2016.

Wikipedia. (2016). "Diagnostic and Statistical Manual of Mental Disorders." Accessed on September 6, 2016.

Wylie, M.S. (2015). "The Limits of Talk: Bessel Van der Kolk Wants to Transform the Treatment of Trauma." www.psychotherapynetworker.org/daily/article/485-the-limits-of-talk/ Accessed on October 5, 2016.

3 Eye Movement Desensitization and Reprocessing

Having stated my contention, and that of most of my colleagues in the field, that "trauma is at the root of the vast majority of mental health diagnoses"; having explored the impact of trauma and memory on the brain; having collected the diverse, contemporary, and staggering statistics that remain; and having explored the controversy around quagmires that can complicate and prohibit the healing of trauma, this chapter focuses on an evidence-based protocol, that when practiced in an *integrated* way, promises to heal the traumatized brain.

Eye Movement Desensitization and Reprocessing (EMDR) has come a long way since Francine Shapiro discovered the potential of bilateral stimulation to calm her anxious thoughts in 1987. In her 2007 article "EMDR, Adaptive Information Processing and Case Conceptualization," Shapiro explains,

> In its 20-year history, it has evolved from a simple technique into an integrative Psychotherapy approach with a theoretical model that emphasizes the brain's information processing system and memories in disturbing experiences as the basis of pathology. The eight-phase treatment comprehensively addresses the experiences that contribute to clinical conditions and those that are needed to bring the client to a robust state of psychological health.
>
> (p. 68)

As Shapiro continues, "This approach is used to process the early memories that set the foundations for the pathology and the present situations that trigger the dysfunction, while providing templates for appropriate future action that incorporate the information and behaviors needed to overcome skill and/or developmental deficits" (p. 68). Shapiro herself provides us with an articulate history of EMDR, which she tells us began in 1989 with a randomized controlled study of trauma victims (p. 68). She dubbed it

> eye movement desensitization, or EMD, because it was informed by a behavioral orientation, and it was thought that eye movements were

unique in causing an effective desensitization. From this vantage point, the treatment effects were viewed primarily as a reduction in the fear and anxiety resulting from the traumatization.

(p. 68)

Over the years, other forms of bilateral stimulation were pinpointed, such as tapping and tones, capable of changing the negative emotions and body sensations of those traumatized into more positive effects, thus creating new behaviors, "a new sense of self." This establishes a neurobiological component to EMDR (Shapiro, 2007).

The neurobiological components of EMDR are patterns of alternating, bilateral stimulation (from left to right) of eye movements, (discovered by Shapiro, mentioned above, and further addressed by Shapiro below), auditory/tactile tones, and bilateral tapping that cause clients' attention to shift back and forth, thereby activating significant brain mechanisms. These components have been further addressed in Robert Stickgold's 2002 article "EMDR: A Putative Neurobiological Mechanism of Action." This author proposes "that the repetitive redirecting of attention in EMDR induces a neurobiological state, similar to that of REM sleep, which is optimally configured to support the cortical integration of traumatic memories into general somatic networks" (p. 61). Stickgold also suggests "that this integration can then lead to a reduction in the strength of hippocampally mediated episodic memories of the traumatic event as well as the memories' associated, amygdala-dependent, negative affect" (p. 61). The integration of memories is a crucial part of the EMDR process. Those who suffer from psychological trauma experience fragmented memories (that lead to an inability to process traumatic episodes), intrusive thoughts, and somatic complaints (see Chapter 1). Furthermore, according to Stickgold, "progress cannot be made with the PTSD patient until she is able to discuss the traumatic event without replaying the episodic memory with its sensory and affective intensity" (p. 69). "Only when these images are no longer intrusive," continues Stickgold, "can she integrate the event into her life, come to understand it, discover what it means for her, and thereby come to terms with it" (p. 69).

A complete discussion of Stickgold's model which, as the author admits, parallels Shapiro's thinking, is beyond the purview of this book (see Stickgold, 2002). However, I feel that it is crucial to highlight the major premise of his model. It is important to affirm Stickgold's goal in his article, "to demonstrate that there is a reasonable explanation of how EMDR works, which is consonant with modern neurobiology and cognitive neuroscience and which provides a basis for future studies of the mechanism of action of EMDR" (p. 62). It is also important to recognize that Stickgold's model offers an explanation of the "physiological processes of REM sleep-integration of the extracted and abstracted core of episodic memories into cortical, semantic memory networks, unimpeded by intrusive, hippocampal replay of the episodic memories" (p. 69).

Stickgold further proposes "how EMDR might serve to bypass a PTSD-induced breakdown in sleep-dependent memory reprocessing" (p. 62). He suggests that

> by inducing neurophysiological and neurochemical changes during the therapeutic session that mimic those seen in REM sleep, the effective integration of traumatic episodic memories into semantic memory networks is achieved. As a consequence, the hippocampal episodic memories and associated affect are believed to be weakened or eliminated, leading to the alleviation of the symptoms of [psychological trauma].
>
> (p. 62)

Obvious advantages of EMDR over what occurs during REM sleep are that our clients are awake and aware of the episodic memories and that an EMDR therapist can help our clients "feel safe" thus minimizing the negative emotions such as fear and anxiety that often occur during the reprocessing of toxic memories (Stickgold, 2002). In the end, what Stickgold dubs the "understanding of the brain basis of EMDR" (p. 72) gives us hope that we can eliminate the divides between neuroscience, psychology, and therapeutic interventions, and thus *integrate* the neural implications and therapeutic protocols in an effort to better heal psychological trauma (see Chapter 6).

Evidence-based Practices

The efficacy of EMDR is unquestionable. When perusing EMDRIA's (the EMDR International Association) website, www.emdria.org, which includes the Francine Shapiro Library, one can only be amazed with the following plethora of information in support of EMDR: 40 randomized controlled studies; 34 non-randomized studies; 8 meta-analyses; 43 articles dealing with the Adaptive Information Processing model and EMDR therapy procedures; 21 randomized controlled studies evaluating the mechanism of the bilateral stimulation component; 25 studies on the hypotheses of eye movements; 23 additional psychophysiological and neurobiological evaluations of EMDR treatment; and 14 studies on the treatment of military personnel. EMDR has proven effective in addressing a multitude of traumas as well as many mental health issues, including addiction, chronic pain, autism, fibromyalgia, hyperactivity, grief, and bi-polar disorder.

While it is beyond the purpose of this book to review the specific contents of EMDR studies that I have mentioned, I encourage my readers to explore EMDRIA's website, www.emdria.org. Ten particular studies published within the last decade, however, resonated with me and warrant a brief summary.

1. The 2007 study "EMDR, Adaptive Information Processing, and Case Conceptualization" was conducted by Francine Shapiro. In her study, Shapiro further defines EMDR as "an integrative, client-centered

psychotherapy approach that emphasizes the brain's information processing system and memories of disturbing experiences as the bases of those pathologies not caused by organic deficit or insult" (p. 68). Next, Shapiro succinctly explains the Adaptive Information Processing (AIP) modality and how it lays the groundwork for and guides clinical practice. As Shapiro comments, "Consistent with neurobiological findings, it is posited that in order to make sense of incoming stimuli, new experiences are assimilated into already existing memory networks" (p. 70). The AIP model posits, continues Shapiro, "that pathology results when unprocessed experiences are stored in their own neural network, unable to link up naturally with anything more adaptive" (p. 70). For example, the person can experience future positive information but, as Shapiro notes, "the new information, positive experiences, and affects are unable to link into the network where the unprocessed material is stored" (p. 70). Using the example of a person suffering from borderline personality disorder who may feel positive about a partner one moment and angry towards them in the next, "The positive experiences are stored in one memory network," notes Shapiro, "but the disturbing experiences of early abandonment or abuse are in another, and can get triggered by anything reminiscent of those events" (p. 70). In sum, according to Shapiro,

> The AIP model distinguishes EMDR from other forms of psychotherapy by viewing the present situations producing distress simply as a trigger for a past, unprocessed incident. It is thought that the current event stimulates the memory network, causing stored negative emotions, physical sensations, and perspectives to emerge.
>
> (p. 71)
>
> Although originally crafted as an individual therapy, Shapiro's case study uniquely demonstrates the merits of EMDR for family systems therapists by guiding her readers through the eight-phase treatment approach to "explore and process the negative experiences that are contributing to dysfunction, and the positive experiences that are needed to bring the client full health."
>
> (p. 72)

2. In a small 2002 pilot study, "Comparison of Two Treatments for Traumatic Stress: A Community-Based Study of EMDR and Prolonged Exposure," researchers Ironson, Freund, Strauss, and Williams analyze the data of 22 clients, namely rape and crime victims, from a university-based clinic serving the community comparing the efficacy of EMDR and Prolonged Exposure (PE), a treatment where patients were instructed to recall the trauma memories and feelings vividly in great detail, as if it were happening again. The first three sessions were similar for both treatment groups in that they evaluated baseline symptoms using the Post Traumatic Stress Disorder Symptom Scale (PSS-SR), the Beck's

Depression Inventory (BDI), the Dissociative Experience Scale (DES), employed psychoeducation, breathing exercises, and a "taped relaxation exercise." Participants also received two active sessions where the PE patients were given the instructions for imaginal exposure as described earlier in this paragraph, and the EMDR sessions followed the eight-phase protocol of EMDR. The results proved that both PE and EMDR were effective in reducing depression. In their attempt to determine how many subjects in each treatment group "had improved sufficiently to terminate trauma" (measured as a 70% reduction in PTSD symptoms), the researchers concluded that "there was significantly more improvements after three active sessions with EMDR (7 of 10 participants) as compared to PE (2 of 12 participants)" (Ironson et al., 2002, p. 120). Among the three participants that did not improve considerably after the three active sessions, "two improved with further treatment, and one did not meet the criterion 70% symptom reduction following three additional active sessions." According to the researchers with PE, "at least four (and possibly another three who left before evaluation of the sixth active session) of the 12 enrolled met criterion after being offered six active treatment sessions whereas with EMDR, with no dropouts, 9 of 10 met criterion after being offered six active sessions" (p. 121). In addition, the researchers discovered that "dropout after the first active session was significantly higher for those randomized to treatment with PE (3 of 10 for PE, 0 of 10 for EMDR)" (p. 122). Regarding the Subjective Units of Distress (SUDS) score, they decreased significantly during the first EMDR session, while PE participants became increasingly distraught. The study included the components of good research including randomized controlled design, advanced treatments, standardized measurements, well-articulated targets, and non-biased assessors. At the same time, there were some limitations including the small sample size, the fact that assessments tended to be mostly self-reports, that "assessors who administered the measures were not blind to treatment condition" and that "PE patients reported higher baseline BDI scores" (p. 125). As the researchers indicated, "both PE and EMDR appeared to work well to reduce PTSD symptoms" (p. 126) but "EMDR was more likely to produce a rapid reduction in symptoms," (p. 126) and "EMDR may be better tolerated, as indicated by a lower dropout rate and lower SUDS scores during the initial session, indicating less subjective patient distress" (p. 126).

3. From a different perspective, "EMDR Treatment for Children with PTSD: Results of a Randomized Controlled Trial," a 2007 study conducted by Abdulbaghi Ahmad, Bo Larsson, and Viveka Sundelin-Wahlsten examined "the efficacy of EMDR treatment for children with post-traumatic stress disorder (PTSD) compared with untreated children in a waiting list control group (WLC) participating in a randomized controlled superiority trial (RTC)" (p. 349). The 33 children were selected

from a total of 179 children at a child psychiatric outpatient clinic for traumatized children based on the fact that they met the full criteria for PTSD in the DSM-IV. They were between the ages of 6 and 16 years of age and suffered from PTSD caused by diverse traumatic experiences including: maltreatment; sexual abuse; road accidents; witnessing unnatural deaths; and other types of trauma. The measures used to assess for the traumas included the Genogram, the Harvard-Uppsala Trauma Questionnaire for Children (HUTQ-C), the Diagnostic Interview for Children and Adolescents (DICA), and the Posttraumatic Stress Symptom Scale for Children (PTSS-C Scale), all of which were conducted in semi-structured interviews with both child and caregiver present. Treatment session measures, part of the EMDR protocol, were also used, such as the Subjective Units of Distress (SUD) and the Validity of Positive Cognition (VOC). Seventeen children were randomized to EMDR treatment and sixteen to the WLC group, with eight sessions per week scheduled for both groups. The children in the EMDR group received immediate treatment after being assessed, while the children in the WCL group waited two months before treatment. There were no significant demographic differences found between the two groups. The authors of this study utilized the appropriate research methods such as the chi-square test, the t-test, and ANCOVA for statistical analysis with the revelation that subjects treated with EMDR had significantly lower post-treatment scores than the subjects in the WCL group, especially regarding the re-experiencing of symptoms (i.e., intrusive images, memories, flashbacks, and nightmares), considered to be the pathogenesis of PTSD. Those in the WLC group improved in PTSD-non-treated symptoms, suggesting that a natural healing process might have been the case when no psychopathology had developed. However, the usual limitation suspects must be considered (i.e., small sample size, highly selective sample size, a heterogeneous group, and lack of follow-up of treatment effects). But in the final analysis, despite these limitations, this controlled study demonstrates the efficacy of EMDR in treating children and adolescents (Ahmad et al., 2007).

4. In their 2006 study "Treatment of PTSD by Eye Movement Desensitization Reprocessing (EMDR) Improves Sleep Quality, Quality of Life, and Perception of Stress," Mara Regina Raboni, Segio Tufik, and Deborah Suchecki once again underscore the efficacy of EMDR. According to the researchers, "The purpose of this study was to examine whether EMDR treatment can improve PTSD symptoms, such as sleep, depression, anxiety, and poor quality of life" (p. 508). While sleep disturbances are often considered secondary symptoms of PTSD, they can be horrific for those suffering from trauma, impacting every part of their waking lives. As my readers already know, given the discussion in the beginning of this chapter and according to the researchers here, "Rapid eye movement sleep specifically plays a role in the integration of traumatic and

stressful memories" (p. 509). They further point out that the findings indicate that "sleep symptoms of PTSD are manifested during REM sleep, when most of the information, learning and memories are processed, including stress—and surviving-related emotional material" (p. 509).

Seven patients aged 24–36 years, high school graduates consisting of two males and five females who were assaulted or kidnapped for at least 3 months and presented with sleep complaints were chosen for this study. They were evaluated utilizing the SCID-DSM IV and IES to confirm PTSD. They were also given a psychological evaluation which consisted of the Beck's Depression Inventory and the Coping Strategy Inventory, among others, which were repeated at the end of treatment. A one-way ANOVA method for statistical analysis was used for repeating measures at the start of treatment, after the third EMDR session, and the week following termination. The results included the following: a decrease in depression, anxiety, fatigue, and impact of event, and an increase in sleep quality and efficiency. The researchers concluded that,

> Among the sleep disorders, insomnia and recurrent nightmares are of particular interest, as recall of the traumatic event takes place generating emotional revival and hyperactivity response. When the traumatic memory loses its negative emotional valence, there is a decrease in arousal and, consequently, an improvement of the harmful PTSD symptoms. The increased sleep efficiency and reduction of general, social, and emotional stress are determining factors for the patients to perceive the improvement in their quality of life and well-being.
>
> (Raboni et al., 2006, p. 511)

5. In another 2014 study supporting the efficacy of EMDR, "Eye Movement Desensitization and Reprocessing in Subsyndromal Bipolar Patients with a History of Traumatic Events: A Randomized, Controlled Pilot-Study," Patricia Novo, Ramon Landin-Romero, Joaquim Radua, Victor Vicens, Isabel Fernandez, Francisca Garcia, Edith Pomarol-Clotet, Peter J. McKenna, Francine Shapiro, and Benedict L. Amann bring to our attention that "traumatic events are frequent in bipolar patients and can worsen the cause of the disease" (p. 21). I refer my readers back to my Preface, having experienced this in "real" terms. As I became aware of the multiple traumatic events experienced by my spouse during his early childhood as well as the negative life experiences, including suffering from chronic pain that occurred during his later adult years, and the fact that they were never reprocessed, I realized that my spouse was suffering from complex PTSD comorbid with adult bipolar disorder. He presented with an intense symptomology including: a magnified prevalence for social difficulties; a need to isolate; intense displays of anger toward figures of authority; intense mood swings; anxiety; depression; mania,

which manifested in his abusing substances; establishing a pattern of risky behavior (i.e., spending large amounts of money); and suicidal ideation and gestures, eventually leading to the taking of his own life.

Novo et al. support the contention that "the evidence of negative effects of traumatic events or PTSD on the course of bipolar disorder is robust " (p. 21). The authors recognize the efficacy of EMDR for the treatment of those suffering from this comorbidity when they comment,

> We found a statistically significant mood stabilizing effect for both depressive and (hypo)manic symptoms in unstable bipolar patients at the end of the Eye Movement Desensitization and Reprocessing intervention. We also found that bipolar patients with subsyndromal symptoms, symptoms that are not severe enough for a clinically random diagnosis, treated with Eye Movement Desensitization and Reprocessing improved significantly in terms of trauma-related symptomology as evaluated by the CAPS and the IES.
>
> (p. 25)

Their conclusions were based on working with a treatment group receiving 14 and 18 EMDR sessions over a period of 12 weeks with evaluations performed by a blind rater at baseline after 2, 5, 8, 12, and 24 weeks. While limitations similar to those presented in the last study were apparent, strengths of their trial included randomized controlled design and a complementary matched sample (Novo et al., 2014).

6. Given the multitude of recent horrific mass trauma situations, many of which are noted at the end of Chapter 1 in a 2005 study "EMDR Therapy Following the 9/11 Terrorist Attacks: A Community-Based Intervention Project in New York City," conducted by Steven Silver, Susan Rogers, James Knipe, and Gina Colelli, more than warrants our attention. While there have been several studies evaluating the effectiveness of EMDR in mass trauma events, this is the first study to evaluate the efficacy of EMDR intervention for terrorism of such magnitude in both the immediate aftermath of the attack, and in the longer range. The authors begin by reviewing the efficacy of EMDR in natural disaster settings as well as the efficacy of school-based EMDR interventions supported by the International Society for Traumatic Stress Studies, the Department of Veterans Affairs and Defense, and Division 12 of the American Psychological Association. They proceed to define the participants in this study as "individuals who had lost a loved one or coworker, who were eyewitnesses to the attacks, or who were involved in rescue, body recovery, or clean-up efforts at the World Trade Center" (p. 33). Although a total of 141 individuals "contacted the network," some were not included in the study due to the "complexity of their problems"

such as complex trauma and other more serious mental health disorders. The 65 participants that were included in the study ranged in age from 6 to 65 years old, and 75% of them were women. This group was divided into two groups, those who were seen 2 to 10 weeks after 9/11 and those who were seen 30 to 48 weeks after 9/11. In order to provide a comparison, a cohort group was made up of the first 12 individuals seen after the first group finished treatment. All of the participants in the study were treated from anywhere between 2 to 48 weeks after 9/11. The groups were seen by clinicians who completed or were very close to completing certification from the EMDR International Association (EMDRIA). Assessments instruments used included the Beck's Depression Inventory (BDI), the Beck's Anxiety Inventory (BAI), the Impact of Event Scale—Revised (IES-R), all of which are multiple-item psychometrics with high validity and reliability and were used during pre- and post-treatment. The Subjective Units of Disturbance Scale (SUD), used to measure the current level of the individual's distress, and the Validity of Cognition Scale (VOC), used to record the negative cognition the individuals hold about themselves, were also used and are measures utilized in the EMDR protocol (see also Chapter 4). As Silver et al. reveal, "The major finding of this study was a 50%–61% decrease in average scores of standardized measures of anxiety, depression and PTSD symptoms and an even greater improvement in self-report measures in an average of 4–5 sessions" (p. 37). The researchers also concluded that "the IES-R average dropped to a level well below the cutoff for major impact. As measured by the BDI, on average clients moved from moderate to mild depression; likewise, the BAI showed changes from moderate range to very mild levels" (p. 37).

The study also discovered that individuals in the latter group after 9/11 were suffering from more distress than those who received immediate treatment and that they did not attain the same positive SUD and VOC results before treatment. The lack of a control group, withholding treatment from the wait-list group and the lack of diagnostic measures, such as the DSM-IV, that would have determined how many of the clients met the diagnostic criteria for PTSD, and the lack of program evaluation studies, however, provide proof of some limitations of this study (Silver, Rogers, Knipe, & Colelli, 2005). However, as I have discovered, the possibility of program evaluation studies pose certain problems in community/mass trauma situations (i.e., the presence of community authorities who may unintentionally limit our clinical response to the victims and the inclusion of care providers who have limited training), with the Sandy Hook shooting a case in point (see Appendix 1).

7. Given the fact that many individuals suffering from trauma are also diagnosed with borderline personality disorder (BPD) and often have suffered from early-onset childhood physical and sexual abuse, parental

pathology, and insecure attachment disorders, to name a few, as I have seen in both research and in my practice, the next study, "EMDR in the Treatment of Borderline Personality Disorder," is significant for establishing the efficacy of EMDR. Utilizing a 2006 case study, Susan Brown and Francine Shapiro explain, "Given the significance of childhood abuse and trauma, eye movement desensitization and reprocessing (EMDR), a recognized trauma therapy, may be a reasonable treatment option for BPD" (p. 403). The individual used in their case study presented with panic, anxiety, depression, raging outbursts, insecurity, low self-esteem, and relationship difficulties given the affair between her husband and sister. However, she also suffered from an insecure attachment style with her biological mother who gave her up from birth after three months, only to claim her back in a dramatic court proceeding with her new spouse from her foster parents when she was two and a half years old. In addition, she was sexually abused at the age of 8 by a cousin, experienced ongoing substance-abuse problems within the parental frame which resulted in many violent fights, eventually leaving her home at 18 to marry her current spouse.

In addition, the individual in this case study later learned that whom she thought was her father was actually her step-father and that she had two half-sisters and a brother. These revelations corresponded with the time when she learned about her husband's affair (Brown and Shapiro, 2006).

The individual in this case study was assessed using the Inventory of Self Capacities, a measure for interpersonal conflicts, abandonment concerns, identity impairment, affect control, dysregulation, instability, affect skills deficits, and tension reduction activity. While her pre-treatment scores before EMDR were beyond clinically significant, her post-treatment scores, after 20 sessions of EMDR, and her seven-month follow-up scores were subclinical. Especially noteworthy is the fact that her Subjective Units of Distress (SUD) scores decreased considerably and her negative cognition "I am not safe" was reversed. As the researchers conclude and admit, "Results in this case study indicate that EMDR is a promising treatment for this population. However, further research is needed to identify what portion of the population can be efficiently treated, which may need a modified version of the standard protocols, and what portion may not be good candidates for EMDR" (p. 416).

8. The next study that I have chosen to discuss briefly focuses on the population who first received the diagnosis of PTSD, war veterans/casualties of war. In their 2006 article, "Treating Combat-Related Stress Disorders: A Multiple Case Study Utilizing Eye Movement Desensitization and Reprocessing (EMDR) with Battlefield Casualties from the Iraqi War," Mark C. Russell focuses on the efficacy of EMDR with four combat veterans selected from approximately 1,400 casualties evacuated from the 2003 Iraqi war, 158 of which were given the diagnosis of

combat-related psychological stress. The ward personnel at the evacuation hospital in Rota, Spain, where Russell was stationed, referred four of the most extreme cases to him for treatment (the maximum that could be added to his caseload given other duties). The four cases were all "requesting relief from intrusive symptoms" and all "terrified of returning home." The assessment measures used included the Structural Clinical Interview, based on the Diagnostic and Statistical Manual of Mental Disorders (DSM-IV), the Impact of Events Scale (a 15-item self-report inventory of intrusive and avoidant symptoms), and the SUDS, a standard part of the EMDR protocol that I am sure all my readers are familiar with given the studies described. EMDR was provided in what we would now call an abbreviated form or recent protocol since they were seen within hours or days of arrival at the field hospital. While this article focuses on the detailed treatment and results of the four participants, which I would highly suggest my readers consult, Russell's experience speaks for itself: "The current finding that substantial remediation of symptoms was achieved after only one session in all four treated veterans may indicate a difference between acute and chronic stress, the number of traumatizing memories necessitating treatment, or (as is more likely) a combination of both" (p. 11). As Russell recognizes, "Future research should examine the variables of time since the incident and the number and type of the patient's traumatic memories" (p. 11). As Russell further acknowledges,

> It is possible that once a veteran is psychologically debilitated, his or her susceptibility to additional traumatization increases during the remaining tour of duty. If true, this fact may indicate that more immediate treatment on the front lines and post-evacuation would result in lower attrition and increased retention and unit readiness.
>
> (p. 11)

9. In the 2011 study "The EMDR Protocol for Recent Critical Incidents [EMDR-PREDI]: Application in a Disaster Mental Health Continuum of Care Context," Ignacio Jarrero, Lucina Artigas, and Marilyn Luber reveal, "For more than 10 years, experts have concluded that the psychological casualties of a disaster will outweigh the physical by an estimated 4:1 ratio" (p. 82). We have certainly had evidence for this conclusion since before and after 2011, when this article was written. As researchers define it,

> *Continuum of care* may be thought of as "a stepped progression of health care provided in an increasingly intensified manner. In psychosocial intervention, we see a progression from crisis intervention, we see a progression from crisis intervention to counseling, to psychotherapy, to psychotropic medical practice, and to psychosocial rehabilitation."
>
> (p. 83)

The researchers developed the EMDR-PRECI, a modification of Shapiro's (2001) Recent Traumatic Events Protocol. In this study,

> all fifty-three employees were provided with CMB. Following that intervention, and in accordance with continuum of care principles, an evaluation was conducted to identify those individuals requiring more comprehensive care. These individuals were provided with EMDR-PRECI, in two groups: immediate treatment group and wait-list/delayed treatment group.
>
> (p. 92)

As the researchers of this study continue, "The results indicated that one session of EMDR-PRECI provided significant improvement on measures of posttraumatic stress for both the immediate and waitlist/delayed treatment groups, with results maintained 12-week follow-up" (p. 92). Accordingly, the researchers conclude,

> This study lends support to the view that the EMDR-PRECI can be used effectively with adults as an early intervention in the acute phase of a critical incident posttraumatic response by reducing symptoms of posttraumatic stress and maintaining those effects despite ongoing threat and danger. The possibility of using this modified EMDR protocol as one component of a comprehensive system of post-disaster interventions has important global implications.
>
> (p. 92)

For those of my readers who would like to better understand the differences between the EMDR protocol and the EMDR-PRECI, I recommend perusing the 2015 article "The EMDR Protocol for Recent Critical Incidents (EMDR-PRECI) and Ongoing Traumatic Stress," by Ignacio Jarero and Lucina Artigas.

10. In the final study noted here, "Early EMDR Intervention Following a Community Critical Incident: A Randomized Clinical Trial," conducted by Elan Shapiro and Brurit Laub in 2015, we more than comprehend the importance of early intervention of EMDR. Six weeks after surviving a missile attack in Gaza, 17 subjects were treated with early EMDR, specifically the Recent Traumatic Episode Protocol (R-TEP) (p. 17).

As the authors explain,

> Volunteer EMDR practitioners [from diverse parts of the country] conducted treatment of 2 consecutive days. Participants were randomly allocated to either immediate or waitlist/delayed treatment conditions. Assessments with Impact of Event Scale Revised (IES-R) and the patient Health Questionnaire (PHQ-9) brief depression inventory took place at pre-and posttreatment and at a 3 months follow-up. At 1 week

> posttreatment, the scores of the immediate treatment group were significantly improved on the IES-R compared to the waitlist/delayed treatment group who showed no improvement prior to their treatment. At 3 months follow-up, the results of the IES-R were maintained and there was a significant improvement on the PHQ-9 scores. This pilot study provides preliminary evidence, supporting the efficacy of EMDR R-TEP for reducing posttrauma stress among civilians of hostility, and shows that this model of intervention briefly augmenting local mental health services following large-scale traumatic incidents, using an EMDR intervention on two consecutive days may be effective.
>
> (p. 17)

It is important for my readers also to comprehend the authors' intent regarding the design of the study. According to Shapiro and Laub,

> The design of the study used a waitlist/delayed treatment comparison to control for spontaneous remission (waitlist comparison) and to attempt to a replication of treatment results (immediate vs. delayed treatment). The IES-R scores of the immediately treatment group significantly improved compared to the waitlist (delayed treatment) group, who showed no improvement prior to their treatment. Although these results suggest no effect on the PTSD symptoms from the spontaneous remission during the 1 week period, there may have been subsequent spontaneous remission as four of the nine waitlist/delayed group participants declined and/or dropped out of treatment.
>
> (pp. 17, 24)

While the pilot study indicates that the EMDR R-TEP can reduce stress and depressive symptoms among this population and aid local mental health services, the limitations of this study and the need for future research are obvious and include: the small sample size; limited screening tools; reliance on self-report instruments; lack of additional variables such as intervention timing and the number and intensity of treatment sessions (Shapiro and Laub, 2015).

The EMDR Recent Traumatic Episode Protocol (EMDR R-TEP) is a logically constructed and encompassing trauma protocol that provides guidelines without the additional treatment strategies offered by the EMDR protocol. EMDR R-TEP includes a screening tool, offers a brief intervention potentially offering rapid treatment effects, usually within two to four sessions, and a significant follow-up component without the homework that is part of the EMDR protocol (Shapiro and Laub, 2015).

I feel strongly that while an early EMDR protocol can be beneficial to those suffering from a traumatic experience since it can halt some symptoms before the faulty integration of the memory takes place and provide some safety, coping, and resourcing skills, it should always be followed by the EMDR protocol. However, I refer my readers to Shapiro's and Laub's (2009) article

"The Recent Traumatic Episode Protocol (R-TEP): An Integrative Protocol for Early Intervention (EEI)" for a comprehensive background and description of the full R-TEP protocol.

The confirmation of the efficacy of EMDR in healing a multitude of traumas is also provided by a host of articles written by Bessel van der Kolk, M.D., whose 2014 book *The Body Keeps the Score: Brain, Mind, and Body in the Healing of Trauma* challenges and excites his readers with innovative topics such as neuroscience, body-brain connections, and the understanding of the tyranny of early attachment. Francine Shapiro herself has published nine comprehensive books to date, including one she edited, *EMDR as an Integrated Psychotherapy Approach: Experts of Diverse Orientations Explore the Paradigm Prism* (2002), which features an array of articles by experts in the field who are willing to "step out of the box."

The highest praise for the efficacy of EMDR in the healing of trauma in both the internal and external family systems comes from the endorsement of government agencies and private organizations including: the American Psychological Association; the California Evidence-based Clearinghouse for Child Welfare; Crest; the Center for Behavioral Health Statistics and Quality; the Centers for Disease Control and Prevention; the Department of Health and Human Services; the Department of Veterans Affairs; the Department of Defense; the National Institute of Mental Health; the National Criminal Justice Reference Service; the National Institute on Alcohol Abuse and Alcoholism; the National Center for PTSD; the Substance Abuse and Mental Health Services Administration (SAMHSA) National Registry for Evidence-based Programs and Practices; the National Child Traumatic Stress Network; the United Kingdom Department of Health; and, most importantly, the World Health Organization (WHO) that names EMDR the first line of treatment for trauma and PTSD in 2013 (see Chapter 1).

Core Components: Understanding EMDR Therapy

There is no doubt in this author's mind, and, I hope, in the minds of my readers, that EMDR is an evidence-based psychotherapeutic and, in part, a neurobiological model for treating trauma and PTSD. The Adaptive Information Processing model, for instance, developed by Francine Shapiro as a "working hypothesis" within the EMDR protocol, addresses the neurobiological aspects of the protocol (2001, p. 54). According to Shapiro, the Adaptive Information Processing model, "is offered as a working neurophysiological *hypothesis* because current understanding of brain physiology is not yet sufficient to verify its accuracy." However, as Shapiro explores in her 2001 book *Eye Movement Desensitization and Reprocessing: Basic Principles, Protocols and Procedures*, "The Adaptive Information processing model states that there is an innate physiological system that is designed to transform disturbing input into an adaptive resolution and a psychologically healthy integration" (p. 54).

This suggests that much of the psychopathology is due to maladaptive encoding and the incomplete processing of traumatic events. These problems impair the client's ability to integrate traumatic experiences in an adaptive manner. The time it takes clients to integrate experiences in an adaptive manner is determined by the severity of the trauma, the length of exposure, age, resources, and the strength of their role models.

As Shapiro starts to explain,

> A trauma may disturb the information-processing system, causing perceptions to be stored in state-dependent form and manifested by pronounced symptoms of PTSD. The blocked information processing is thought to be stimulated through a variety of possible physiological factors including (1) deconditioning caused by a complicated relaxation response, (2) a shift in brain state enhancing the activation and strengthening of weak associations, or (3) some other function of a dual-focus information-processing mechanism.
>
> (p. 54)

Shapiro continues,

> the model regards most pathologies as derived from earlier life experiences that set in motion a continued pattern of affect, behavior, cognitions and consequently identity structures. The pathological structure is inherent within the static, insufficiently processed information stored at the time of the disturbing event . . . The continued influence of these early experiences is due in large part to the present-day stimuli eliciting the negative affect and beliefs embodied in these memories and causing the client to continue acting in a way consistent with the earlier events. Although a client's memory may be of an actual event and of behavior that may then have been appropriate for the disturbing situation, the lack of adequate assimilation means that the child is still reacting emotionally and behaviorally in ways consistent with the earlier disturbing incident . . . EMDR processing of such memories allows the more positive and empowering present affect and cognitions to generalize to the associated memories throughout the neurophysiological network and leads spontaneously to more appropriate behaviors in the client.
>
> (pp. 16–17)

In the end, as Shapiro importantly recognizes, "adopting the Adaptive Information Processing model can facilitate the ability of many EMDR-trained clinicians to achieve both substantial and comprehensive treatment effects" (p. 17).

EMDR is constructed around a clearly articulated eight-phase modality developed by Francine Shapiro and summarized according to purpose and procedures that progress through history-taking, assessment, preparation for EMDR treatment, desensitization, installation, body scan, closure, and reevaluation. This author has taken the liberty to present Shapiro's eight-phase modality (see Appendix 2) with subtle alterations that can potentially increase the reach of EMDR treatment.

During Phase One, or the client history-taking phase, the therapist inquires as to what has brought the patient in and the symptoms and behaviors they are experiencing. More specifically, the therapist identifies the client's targets for EMDR, otherwise known as the disturbing events, memories, issues, and feelings of the past and identifies the present situations that have exacerbated them as well as the "maladaptive" beliefs or cognitions that the client has formulated about herself (e.g., "I am not safe"). At this juncture, the therapist obtains the patient's history and a treatment plan is developed.

During Phase Two, the therapist attempts to engage the client in a stabilization process by having the client select an image of a safe/calm place in their lives that encourages pleasant feelings as well as a more positive sense of self in order to help the client face the challenges in Phase Four, when they are engaged in reprocessing the negative events, memories, and body sensations. It is at this point, in Phase Two, that I install this safe/calm place with slow, bilateral stimulation (BLS). According to Shapiro, when a traumatic or distressing experience occurs, it may overwhelm normal coping mechanisms. The memory and associated stimuli are inadequately processed and stored in an isolated memory network. The goal of BLS is to reintegrate the isolated memories into the brain's normal memory. Instead of having the client follow a moving object such as the therapist's fingers or a light bar from side to side with her eyes, however, I use the Advanced TAC/Audi Scan developed by Neuro-Tack Corporation, an audio and tactile device that offers the same bilateral component, but without distractions and headaches that can result when using the former tools. Since "client trust" is extremely important in this phase, as in every phase, I implement a psychoeducational component that explains the EMDR process that increases my client's level of comfort. Establishing a safe environment is especially important when working with those who suffer from childhood trauma. In his 2003 article, "The Neurobiology of Childhood Trauma and Abuse," van der Kolk explains, "Clinical experience shows that children are unlikely to give up their primitive self-protective behaviors until they learn how to feel physically competent and secure. Actual experience with safety and predictability is essential to establish the capacity to regulate physiologic arousal that is indispensable for observing what is going on, process the information, and initiate the appropriate motor responses (i.e., for the establishment of executive functioning)" (p. 310).

During Phase Three, clients are encouraged to identify an image that relates to the disturbing target as well as the negative cognition (NC), a negative belief about herself that arises when facing the target (see Appendix 3). A positive cognition is also determined by the client during this phase.

In Phase Four, the desensitization phase, the therapist encourages the client to focus on the target image selected, the negative cognition (e.g., "I am not safe"), disturbing emotions, and body sensations. The client is then asked what her level of disturbance is around that target, cognition, emotions, and bodily sensations. This is assessed by using the Subjective Units of Disturbance Scale (SUD) based on a scale of 1–10, with 10 being the worst. After completing a set of audio and tactile BLS, clients are asked, "Where did you go?" This translates into "What image, thought, feeling, memory or physical sensation came up for you?" The therapist completes another set of BLS and asks the client the same questions. The number of sets of BLS is determined by the severity and repetitive nature of the target memory. During the desensitization process, the therapist will often inquire about the client's current level of distress or SUD. The desensitization phase is complete only when the client has reached a SUD of 0 or 1. Often during this phase a client will get "stuck," and a cognitive interweave is used to open the blocked issue. Cognitive Interweaves are brief strategies, particularly the use of questions, intended to change the client's perspective in order to allow them to keep processing. Cognitive Interweaves are often indicated when matters arise about clients' defectiveness, safety, or choice (e.g., "The abuse was my fault"; "I should have stopped him from killing himself"; "His suicide was my fault"; or "I put myself in the line of danger, it is my fault.").

In Phase Five, the Installation Phase, the therapist tries to determine whether the positive cognition has changed. If the client's negative cognition was "I am not safe," the therapist identifies the Validity of the positive Cognition (VOC) by asking whether the client feels safe and "How valid does the PC feel, on a scale of 1–7" with a score of 7 indicating that the PC is true. Support and the provision of new skills may be necessitated at this juncture if the client has not reached a VOC of 7.

In Phase Six, a body scan of the client is conducted. The client is asked if they are experiencing any residual pain, discomfort, or stress in any part of the body. If they are experiencing any residuals, additional sets of BLS are performed until the client reports "a clear body scan."

To the drumbeat of emphasis upon the importance of physical responses to psychological trauma provided by Francine Shapiro's somatic focus and Bessel van der Kolk's dictum that "the body keeps the score," we can add, still within Phase Six, the contribution of Stephen Porges' polyvagal theory (Porges, 2011). "Polyvagal" refers to the multiple (specifically, three) roles of the vagal nerve. That nerve is the 10th cranial nerve and the body's second largest and travels from the brain stem all the way to the stomach, so that it can affect a host of the body's components, from the heart to the face. As Porges explains in his 2010 book *The Polyvagal Theory*, "The vagus is not a single neural pathway, but rather a complex bidirectional system with myelinated branches linking the brainstem and various target organs. These neural pathways allow direct and rapid communication between brain structures and specific organs" (p. 135). Porges continues,

> The polyvagal theory proposes that the evolution of the mammalian automatic nervous system provides the neurophysiological substrates for

adaptive behavioral strategies. It further proposes that physiological state limits the range of behavioral and psychological experience. The theory links the evolution of the autonomic nervous system to affective experience, emotional expression, facial gestures, vocal communication and contingent social behavior.

(p. 59)

The three particular responses to which Porges calls our attention are tied to three stages of our evolutionary history, reaching back to our reptilian past and ending with our fully mammalian proclivity to sociality.

The evolutionarily earliest response in our suite of three is the tendency to freeze or become immobilized in the presence of a perceived threat. This is most familiar to us in what we often call an animal's "playing dead" while in the jaws of a predator. Human beings can display this response, too, as in Porges' example of a woman who fainted on a plane that was coming in for a precarious and potentially deadly landing. It is important to recognize that this most primitive bodily response to perceived deadly danger, along with the other two, is not a conscious decision but rather a subliminal, somatic one. Porges coins the term "neuroception" to designate this unique mechanism for reacting to danger.

The second of the responses is more familiar to most of us: the fight-or-flight response in which our body ramps up for action via, for example, adrenalin pouring into the bloodstream and an increased heart rate. While this response, like the previous one, has been essential for the survival of numerous species including our own down through the history of evolution, it should be evident that it is extraordinarily problematic for a trauma survivor to have these responses arise again and again as he or she goes through life encountering triggers that take him or her back to their trauma.

The third vagal response is the least well known but arguably the most important, namely, the social communication and engagement response, a function of the "social nervous system." This response brings us home to the psychologically safe place that is our immediate human community. Arielle Schwartz explains the significance of this by noting that

> Our natural state of rest and safety allows us to engage our social nervous system facilitating our ability to connect to others, feel playful, feel love, and relax into connection. When we experience threat we will initially attempt to use our social nervous system to re-establish connection and safety. For example, 'tend and befriend' behaviors are a stress response that attempts to re-establish a safe relational bond.
>
> (Schwartz, 2014)

"The polyvagal theory of emotions," as van der Kolk points out in his Foreword in Porges's *The Polyvagal Theory,* "has had a profound effect on helping us organize the treatment of abused children and traumatized adults" (p. xv;

see Chapter 16 in *The Polyvagal Theory*, 2010). As Porges carefully summarizes the matter,

> When there are no challenging environmental demands, the automatic nervous system, through the vagus, services the needs of the internal viscera to enhance growth and restoration. However in response to environmental demands, homeostatic processes are compromised, and the automatic nervous system supports increased metabolic output to deal with these external challenges by vagal withdrawal and sympathetic excitation. By mediating the distribution of resources, the central nervous system regulates the strength and latency of automatic responses to deal with internal and external demands.
> (p. 137; see also *The Polyvagal Theory*, pp. 133–134)

Arielle Schwartz offers concrete practices that can bring this social nervous system into play when one is feeling anxiety, panic, or depression, symptoms frequently associated with trauma:

- Focus on the present moment
- Engage the sense of smell with an essential oil that brings a positive association or feeling
- Re-establish connection by calling a friend, snuggling with your pet, or loving self-touch
- Express feelings through talking, writing, drawing, movement
- Focus on your breath as a fine tuning [sic] mechanism to regulate the nervous system
- Engage in a mindfulness practice such as meditation or therapeutic yoga
- Allow yourself to play

(Schwartz, 2014)

The reader will immediately note the many ways in which this application of polyvagal theory to trauma overlaps with material that we have already explored and will continue to explore in this text.

Phase Seven, known as the debriefing component of EMDR treatment, should be implemented after every desensitization session. It focuses on providing the client with support and appropriate information as to what they might expect between sessions and recommending the technique of journaling should they experience any residuals that would impact their safety and stabilization. If residuals are encountered, the therapist should further enhance self-control techniques.

Finally in Phase Eight, the re-evaluation phase, the client is asked by the therapist to report on any new experiences or levels of disturbance arising from previous sessions with the objective that all relevant historical traumas have been processed. Since every client is different with regard to their history, attachment style, diagnoses, and number and severity of their traumas, one is unlikely to be able to predict the number of sessions in this Eight-Phase process (see Appendix 3).

EMDR also involves a three-pronged process to integrate information. This process results in the alleviation of earlier experiences, the recognition of current situations that trigger these disturbances, and provides skills and education to deal with potential future challenges, thus allowing clients suffering from trauma to thrive. The EMDR protocol improves one's sense of self or positive cognition and can improve negative somatic experiences. EMDR utilizes a comprehensive treatment with a unique standard set of procedures and clinical protocols. It incorporates (1) client stability, (2) dual focus of attention, and (3) alternating visual, auditory, and/or tactile stimulation. This process is effective because, as memory research suggests, memories are fluid and can be changed.

The Role of the EMDR Therapist

In his 2010 book *In an Unspoken Voice: How the Body Releases Trauma and Restores Goodness*, Peter A. Levine captures the essence of the role of the EMDR therapist as one who "help[s] to create an environment of *relative* safety, an atmosphere that conveys refuge, hope and possibility. But pure empathy and a warm therapeutic atmosphere are not enough, for traumatized people are often unable to fully read or fully receive compassion" (p. xi).

As Gabor Mate writes in his Forward in Levine's book,

> So what is the therapist to do with human beings hurt and beaten down by trauma? It is to help people listen to the unspoken voice of their own bodies and to enable them to feel their 'survival emotions' of rage and terror without being overwhelmed by these powerful states.
>
> (p. xi)

As Levine himself puts it, "In the therapy situation, the therapist must strike a balance between mirroring a client's distress enough for them to learn about the client's sensations, but not so much as to increase the client's level of fear as in contagion panic" (pp. 46–47).

"This can only happen," continues Levine, "if the therapist has learned the ins and outs of his or her own sensations and emotions and is relatively comfortable with them" (p. 47). Levine also recognizes the importance of addressing what happens in the body during trauma and the therapist's role in aiding and tracking the client "to recognize the psychoemotional and physical signs of 'frozen trauma' in the client. He or she must learn to hear the 'unspoken voice' of the body so that clients can safely learn to hear and see themselves" (p. xii).

In his Foreword in Porges' *The Polyvagal Theory*, van der Kolk brings back the importance of the polyvagal theory in keeping our clients safe. As he notes,

> It is difficult to trace all the sources of one's inspiration, but Porges polyvagal theory gave us a powerful means of understanding how both bodily

states and mental constructs dynamically interact with environmental triggers to precipitate maladaptive behaviors. Porges helps us to understand how dynamic our biological systems are and gave us an explanation why a kind face and a soothing tone of voice can dramatically alter the entire organization of the human organism—that is how being seen and understood can help shift people out of disorganized and fearful states.

(p. xvi)

In a 2012 *New York Times Blog*, "Expert Answers on E.M.D.R," which I encourage my readers to consult, Francine Shapiro elegantly addresses the all-important practical role of the EMDR therapist training: "E.M.D.R. therapy is taught only to people who are licensed to provide mental health services in their state." Shapiro continues,

> major memory processing with E.M.D.R. therapy should be conducted only by a licensed therapist who has had training approved by the EMDR International Association (www.emdria.org), an independent professional association that sets the standards for all E.M.D.R. therapy training conducted in the United States. Comparable organizations exist in most countries worldwide, as well as regional organizations like E.M.D.R. Europe (www.emdr-europe.org), E.M.D.R. Asia (www.emdr-asia.org) and E.M.D.R. Iberoamerica (emdriberoamerica.org).

Shapiro reinforces the point that sufficient training in any therapeutic technique is ethically required. There are substandard versions of EMDR treatment offered at some places in the United States, and persons seeking EMDR ought to investigate therapists' levels of training and their success rate.

Having obtained certification in EMDR approved by the E.M.D.R. International Association (EMDRIA) has proved invaluable for me when working with those suffering from intense and complex psychological trauma. I often encounter individuals and couples, however, who have worked with therapists practicing EMDR who only completed the introductory courses and have just begun to work with this population. Almost four years later, these individuals and couples are still suffering from the specter of trauma. This is the reason why I feel very strongly that in order to really understand the EMDR protocol, and how it can help trauma survivors to "get their lives back," one should continue training beyond the introductory courses and become an EMDRIA certified EMDR clinician. This process, for example, requires many more client contact hours, additional supervision, and continuing education credits, a process which takes approximately two years to complete.

Simply for the sake of completeness, and given our interest in the neurological dynamics involved in treating trauma, it is worth briefly mentioning another matter with potentially important implications for the therapist's unique role with clients, namely, that a large proportion of both neuroscientists and philosophers of mind today deny the reality of what we ordinarily mean by "free will." Although we all have an immediate sense that our actions are, barring the proverbial gun to our heads, under the control of our unique, individual consciousness, some researchers hold that both contemporary experiments and careful analysis of the notion of free will proves it to be an illusion (Harris, 2012).

In addressing the role of the therapist, it might be illuminating to consider the implications of free will for therapy. One might initially suppose that the implications would be devastating. How can the therapist help clients if she or he comes to believe that those clients have no free will to which one can appeal? While we do not have space here to examine the details of this issue, suffice it to say that the current contentions about our lack of free will do not have significant implications for therapeutic practice, whether in the treatment of trauma or in the attempt to alleviate other problems. First of all, even if we are all "determined" by a host of causes, from genetics and brain chemistry to environmental formation, we each act in a way that is a function of our own unique set of such causes or inputs. I act in a way that is determined by who I am, not who you are. This ends up, from a practical perspective, being very similar to what has usually been meant by free will (this way of harmonizing determinism with the traditional concept of free will is known as "compatibilism").

Furthermore, the therapist's interventions are, from the perspective of those who deny free will, still an input into the menagerie of factors that supposedly determine a client's behavior. As such, those interventions can be expected to have precisely the same effects as interventions in a context where clients are believed to have free will. In the end, then, therapists need not lose sleep over contemporary discussions of "free will versus determinism" in scientific and philosophical circles (for an overview of these discussions, see Harris, 2012).

The Postmodern Paradigm granted family therapists global permission to accept the all-important "collaborative" therapeutic relationship in which client and therapist are mutually involved in a compassionate journey of self-discovery in which primary emphasis is placed on understanding the client's experiences. The effects of such a collaborative journey are most positive in the healing of abuse, violence, and trauma on different levels of family experiences (see Mille and Torres, 2009). The client-therapist relationship is crucial in all phases of the Eight Phases of EMDR. Many clients suffering from trauma have been in therapy before without much success. It is especially important for these clients to feel the positive effects of psychoeducation, to feel safe, connected, adequately paced in their treatment, and to feel a sense of equanimity around the process. In his 2003 article "The Neurobiology of Childhood Trauma and Abuse," van der Kolk eloquently summarizes the role of the therapist when working with children,

> The task of therapy is to help these children develop a sense of physical mastery and awareness of who they are and what has happened to them to learn to observe what is happening in the present time and physically

respond to the current demands instead of recreating the traumatic past behaviorally, emotionally and biologically.

(p. 311)

Finally, I believe that it is critical for trauma clinicians to keep current with research and evidence-based practice (keeping in mind that it often takes a number of years to translate research findings into practice), and integrate these components with their clinical practice.

In the next chapter, I shall expand upon this clearly articulated Eight Phase modality using a more inclusive, integrated, and diverse lens in an effort to enhance the EMDR protocol. I feel strongly that the history, preparation, and assessment phases of EMDR treatment are crucial in healing psychological trauma within the systems paradigm and require *mindfulness*, flexibility, and a special kind of finesse regarding the following: psychoeducation; history-taking; identifying targets, current triggers, goals, and suitability for treatment; utilizing a comprehensive and diverse range of evidence-based intake, screening and diagnostic tools; recognizing secure or insecure attachment styles; the presence of dissociation; addressing the individual's Internal Family Systems (IFS) and external family systems; and utilizing additional diverse, safe, and creative stabilizing techniques and resources.

Another topic that requires attention in this chapter is dissociation. In *The Body Keeps the Score: Brain, Mind, and Body in the Healing of Trauma*, (2014), van der Kolk recognizes the critical role of dissociation when addressing traumas:

Dissociation is the essence of trauma. The overwhelming experience is split off and fragmented, so that the emotions, sounds, images, thoughts, and physical sensations related to the trauma take on a life of their own. The sensory fragments of memory, intrude into the present, where they are literally relived.

(p. 66)

Thus, the disruption of ordinarily well-put together functions of a conscious mind, memory, and perceptions which creates intense fragmentation, hypervigilance, irrational emotional overload, flashbacks, and negative somatic sensations must be addressed early on in the EMDR protocol.

Van der Kolk, for example, devotes an entire chapter to "Putting the Pieces Together: Self-Leadership," in his 2014 book *The Body Keeps the Score: Brain, Mind, and Body in the Healing of Trauma*, where he advocates for the importance of "ego state" work by employing the Internal Family Systems (IFS) model. Thus the implications for healing trauma in the systems paradigm by utilizing aspects of the IFS will also be more closely considered in the next chapter.

In addition, attachment styles will be covered in the next chapter since attachment is the connection established early in one's life. It helps a child understand how to control thoughts and emotions. If the child's needs are met, the attachment will be secure. If their needs are not met, however, the attachment will most likely be insecure, producing an inability to self-regulate thoughts and emotions and connect with others in a healthy and functional way. This inability to self-regulate and connect with others can lead to dissociation, a state of being expressed in the development of separate personality parts, a negative sense of self, and memories that are not realized as accurate, an unintegrated 'self,' thus threatening the ability to enhance the EMDR protocol.

As for the next task, since research recognizes EMDR as a protocol with neurobiological aspects, namely the bilateral stimulation component, this author feels compelled to explore other trauma-based treatments that have neurological underpinnings and brain stimulating techniques and examine how these techniques compare with EMDR in terms of efficacy. As we have seen earlier in this chapter, the EMDR protocol has demonstrated efficacy in providing relief to those suffering from psychological traumas, but I have spent little time here on neural explanation. In his 2010 article, "EMDR's Neurobiological Mechanisms of Action: On the Survey of 20 Years of Searching," however, Uri Bergmann summarizes several neuroimaging studies after EMDR including: left frontal lobe activation; decreased occipital activation and decreased temporal lobe activation indicating emotional regulation because of the increased activity of the prefrontal lobe; inhibition of limbic over-stimulation by increasing regulation of the association cortex; reduction in the intrusive and over-consolidating traumatic episodic memory; the reduction of occipitally mediated flashbacks; and the induction of a functions balance between the limbic and prefrontal areas (Bergmann, 2010).

In their 2009 article, "On the Neural Base of EMDR Therapy: Insights from (qEEG) Studies," Melvin L. Harper, Tasha Rasolkhani-Kalhorn, and John F. Drozd also consider the neural possibilities in healing trauma. These authors, for example, after exploring the qEEG or quantitative electro-encephalogram, report,

> the neural basis for the EMDR effect is depotentiation of fear memory synapses in the amygdala during an evoked brain state similar to that of slow wave sleep. These studies suggest that brain stimulation during EMDR significantly increases the power of a naturally occurring low-frequency rhythm in memory areas of the brain, binding these areas together and causing receptors on the synapses of fear memory traces to be disabled. This mechanical change in the memory trace enables it to be incorporated into the normal memory system without the extreme emotions previously associated with it. EMDR is a medical [neurobiological] procedure because it changes the physical structures of the brain to modify problematic stored memories.
>
> (p. 81)

In her 2015 posting "The Limits of Talk: Bessel van der Kolk Wants to Transform the Treatment of Trauma," on *Psychotherapy Networker*, Mary Sykes Wylie refers to van der Kolk's 1994 paper "The Body Keeps the Score," where he explores current research about how neurobiology underlies trauma. As Wylie explains,

> The paper described how trauma disrupts the stress-hormone system, plays havoc with the entire nervous system, and keeps people from processing and integrating trauma memories into conscious mental frameworks. Because of these complex physiological processes, van der Kolk explained in the paper, traumatic memories, in effect, stay "stuck" in the brain's nether regions—the nonverbal, nonconscious, subcortical regions (amygdala, thalamus, hippocampus, hypothalamus, and brain stem), where they are not accessible to the frontal lobes—the understanding, thinking, reasoning parts of the brain.

In his 2008 interview "Bessel van der Kolk on Trauma, Development and Healing," posted on *psychotherapy.net*, David Bullard tells us van der Kolk's reaction to another neurobiological treatment strategy known as neurofeedback: "In neurofeedback," comments van der Kolk, "you change your brain's electrical activity by playing computer games with your own brain waves. Learning how to interpret quantitative EEG's helped me to visualize better how the brain processes information, and how disorganized the brain becomes in response to trauma."

Furthermore, says van der Kolk,

> Learning how to interpret quantitative EEG's [in the content of neurofeedback] allowed me to visualize what parts of the brain are distorted by traumatic experiences, and this can help us target specific areas of the brain where there is abnormal activity and where the problem actually is. For example, for the part of the brain supposed to be in charge, after trauma it will have excessive activity, keeping people in a state of chronic arousal—making it difficult to sleep, hard to engage and to relax. We find neurofeedback can change the activity in parts of the brain to allow it to be more calm and self-observant.
>
> (p. 8)

Utilizing neurofeedback as a means of normalizing electrical regulatory patterns, with the goal of calming the central nervous system and decreasing the symptoms associated with trauma, will be further explored in Appendix 4 by my colleagues Jeffrey J. Schutz, Owner and Executive Director, and Lindsay K. Higdon, Clinical Director of Neurofeedback Services, at The Neurovation Center in Sandy Hook, Connecticut.

At this juncture, this author would like to briefly summarize other neural "brain stimulating techniques" that are more controversial but that have captured the attention of clinicians, researchers, and most importantly, those suffering from trauma, such as electroconvulsive therapy (ECT), EFT Tapping, Brainspotting, and Transcranial Magnetic Stimulation.

In her August 2016 article "Can Tainted Treatment Make a Shock Return?" Jessica Hamzelou thoroughly considers the effects of ECT. ECT, or "shock therapy," was introduced in 1938 by Italian neurologists Ugo Cerletti and Lucio Bini as a treatment for psychosis. The procedure as done before the mid-1950s, attaching electrodes to a patient's head with electrical current passed between them, was damaging to patients' overall brain health . Even so, ECT has been used as a treatment for many mental health conditions since the 1930s by delivering "a jolt of electricity to the brain that triggers a seizure" (p. 16). While the original procedure took place in a hospital operating room where recipients were given a muscle relaxant and general anesthetic, ECT is now used in a routine out-patient environment. However, it remains an uncomfortable procedure, induces a seizure, adds the risk of general anesthesia, and results in confusion and short-term memory problems, and even permanent memory loss in some cases. The use of ECT seems to alter chemicals in the brain in depression, bi-polar, and anxiety-related disorders. ECT appears to have the same effect as antidepressant drugs that heighten the activity of serotonin and dopamine in the brain (Hamzelou, 2016). As Hamzelou further explains,

> There is plenty of evidence that ECT triggers the release of a protein called brain-derived neurotrophic factor, too. This protein spurs the growth and development of new brain cells—a process that happens in healthy brains, but is halted in conditions like depression and schizophrenia. The higher the levels of the protein after ECT, the better the remission of depression. And brain regions that appear shrunken in depression—areas involved in emotion and memory—increase in size after ECT.
>
> (p. 16)

"But ECT," continues Hamzelou, "is pretty extreme . . . and it is usual to have headache, jaw pain and mild confusion for a while after treatment. Short-term memory problems are common and a small percentage of people report permanently losing memories of events from around the time of their treatment" (p. 17). Many trials demonstrate that ECT can be effective for the treatment of short-term depression. But the level and permanency of cognitive impairments and exactly how it should be utilized have been neglected in the randomized controlled studies according to the UK's National Institute for Health and Care Excellence. While the US Food and Drug Administration (FDA) advocates making this technique more accessible for patients suffering from depression and bi-polar disorders, a 2005 study in Switzerland reports only 1% of psychiatrists are in favor of ECT, and 56% are against ECT (Hamzelou, 2016).

Brainspotting, introduced by David Grand from International University and first taught by Grand in 2009, is used by many therapists in diverse countries to treat those suffering from war trauma and community disasters, to name a few. Those practicing Brainspotting maintain that when tapping on the face, hands, and upper body, there is an increased flow of information to the brain and the nervous system which has the potential to calm the amygdala, an important part of the brain's limbic system, an emotional part of the brain associated with hyperarousal and many other symptoms in clients who suffer from trauma. Supporters of Emotional Freedom Techniques (EFT), or tapping, also point to the work of Stephen Porges and his work on the Polyvagal Theory, which suggested that effective tapping can stimulate the most advanced part of the vagus nerve and help the patient feel calm and safe. Since neuroplasticity is the brain's way of changing how thoughts, memories, and sensations are processed, this may explain how EFT's tapping could work in healing trauma. However, according to Brandon A. Gaudiano and James D. Herbert in their August 2000 article "Can We Really Tap Our Problems Away? A Critical Analysis of Thought Field Therapy," in the magazine *Skeptical Inquirer*, "Thought Field Therapy is marketed as an extraordinary fast and effective body-tapping treatment for a number of psychological problems [including trauma]. However it lacks even basic empirical support and exhibits many of the trappings of a pseudoscience" (p. 1).

During Brainspotting, therapists guide clients to "position their eyes" to "target sources of negative emotion." Using a pointer, therapists help clients to slowly follow their eyes across a determined "field of vision" to locate a brainspot, "an eye position that calls up a traumatic memory or painful emotion." It is believed that by engaging in this process, therapists can locate emotions on a deep level and "target the physical effects of trauma." Brainspotting is claimed to "activate the body's innate ability to heal itself from trauma." Some practitioners believe that "Brainspotting works primarily on the limbic system, a collection of brain structures that play a role in emotions, long-term memory, cognition, motivation, impulse control and several other psychological factors that can affect well-being" ("Brainspotting", 2016, p. 1). Though many therapists report positive results from utilizing Brainspotting, this is one of the newer neural approaches, thus further research is needed since few studies have been done on Brainspotting, and it is not as well supported as neural practices previously mentioned.

Grand has also used BioLateral Sound CDs. BioLateral sounds including those from nature and music are used as an alternative to eye movements as a form of bilateral stimulation. While Grand has been given permission by EMDRIA to teach a Distance Learning Program in "Natural Flow EMDR," a model drawing from somatic experience, body resourcing, and ego state work, EMDRIA has not yet taken a stand one way or the other on its efficacy, due to the lack of evidence-based research.

After attending a recent EMDRIA presentation on Mindfulness and EMDR offered by Irene Siegel, I was exposed to Grand's CDs. After purchasing one of them, I discovered that it allowed some of my trauma clients suffering from high-beta brain wave activity to lower their stress more rapidly during EMDR, perhaps due to tranquil, low-frequency SUDS reprocessing offered by the CDs. This, however, requires the research of my neurofeedback colleagues at my practice and, as such, is beyond the purview of my book.

There is another important connection between music and my clients. As Stephan Porges notes in his 2010 book *The Polyvagal Theory*, "Music in the frequency band of human voice, however, elicits visceral and emotional states that are associated with neither impending doom nor a sense of urgency. As such," continues Porges, "music in the frequency band of human voice is often used melodically in compositions to convey the functional and metaphorical 'voice' of the composer" (p. 247). As Porges summarizes his thinking,

> Based on the polyvagal theory, elements of music therapy can be deconstructed into biobehavioral processes that stimulate social engagement system. When the social engagement system is stimulated, the client responds both behaviorally and physiologically. First, the observable features of social engagement become more spontaneous and contingent as the face and voice become more expressive. Second, there is a change in physiological state regulation that is expressed through increased behavioral regulation and calmness. The improved state regulation is mediated by the myelinated vagus, which directly promotes health, growth, and restoration. However, for some clients, especially those who have been traumatized, face-to-face interventions can be threatening and may not elicit a neuroception of safety. In these circumstances, the social engagement system can potentially be activated through vocal prosody or music while minimizing direct face-to-face interactions.
>
> (p. 253)

As for another tool, according to the Mayo Clinic (2015),

> Transcranial Magnetic Stimulation (TMS) is a noninvasive procedure that uses magnetic fields to stimulate nerve cells in the brain to improve symptoms of depression. TMS is typically used when other depression treatments haven't been effective. During a TMS session, an electromagnetic coil is placed against your scalp near your forehead. The electromagnet painlessly delivers a magnetic pulse that stimulates nerve cells in the region of your brain involved in mood control and depression. And it might activate regions of the brain that have decreased activity in people with depression.
>
> (p. 1)

Another 2014 internet posting by the Canadian Agency for Drugs and Technologies in Health, "Transcranial Magnetic Stimulation for the Treatment of Adults with PTSD, GAD, or Depression: A Review of Clinical Effectiveness and Guidelines," reports:

Clinically brain stimulation has been found to improve symptoms of depression, however due to the multifactorial nature of the intervention, the overall effectiveness of TSM for the treatment of depression remains unclear. Even less well known is the efficacy and effectiveness of TMS for the treatment of PTSD and GAD.

(p. 1)

In the next chapter, I will lay the integrative groundwork for enhancing the EMDR protocol. This will further illuminate the value of the information covered in the previous chapters. We shall be on our way to a truly multifaceted, integrated EMDR practice.

References

Ahmad, A., Larsson, B., & Sundelin-Walsten, V. (2007). "EMDR Treatment for Children with PTSD: Results of a Randomized Controlled Trial." *Nordic Journal of Psychiatry*, 61 (5), 349–354.

Bergmann, U. (2010). "EMDR's Neurobiological Mechanisms of Action: On the Survey of 20 Years of Searching." *Journal of EMDR Practice and Research*, 4, 22–42.

"Brainspotting." (2016). *Good Therapy.org*. www.goodtherapy.org/learn-about-therapy/types/brainspottingtherapy#HowDoesBrainspottingWork? Accessed on December 12, 2016.

Brown, S., & Shapiro, F. (2006). "EMDR in the Treatment of Borderline Personality Disorder." *Clinical Case Studies*, 5 (5), 403–420.

Bullard, D. (2014). "Bessel van der Kolk on Trauma, Development and Healing." www.psychotherapy.net/interview/bessel-van-der-kolk-trauma Accessed on October 5, 2016.

E.M.D.R. Asia. www.emdr-asia.org

E.M.D.R. Europe. www.endr-europe.org

E.M.D.R. International Association. www.emdria.org

Gaudiano, B.A., & Herbert, J.D. (2000). "Can We Really Tap Our Problems Away? A Critical Analysis of Thought Field Therapy." *Skeptical Inquirer*, 24. www.csicop.org

Hamzelou, J. (2016). "Can Tainted Treatment Make a Shock Return?" *New Scientist*, 231, 16–17.

Harper, M.L., Rasolkhani-Kalhorn, T., & Drozd, T. (2009). "On the Neural Basis of EMDR Therapy: Insights from QEEG Studies." *Traumatology*, 15, 81–95.

Harris, S. (2012). *Free Will*. New York: Simon and Schuster.

Ironson, G., Freund, B., Strauss, J.L., & Williams, J. (2002). "Comparison of Two Treatments for Traumatic Stress: A Community-Based Study of EMDR and Prolonged Exposure." *Journal of Clinical Psychology*, 58 (1), 113–128.

Jarrero, I., & Artigas, L. (2015). "The EMDR Protocol for Recent Critical Incidents (EMDR-PRECI) and Ongoing Traumatic Stress." emdrresearchfoundation.org/toolkit/preci.pdf Accessed on November 5, 2016.

Jarrero, I., Artigas, L., & Luber, M. (2011). "The EMDR Protocol for Recent Critical Incidents: Application in a Disaster Mental Health Continuum of Care Context." *Journal of Practice and Research*, 5 (3), 82–94.

Levine, P.A. (2010). *In an Unspoken Voice: How the Body Releases Trauma and Restores Goodness.* Berkeley, CA: North Atlantic Books.

Mille, D., & Torres, B.A. (2009). "The Client-Therapist Relationship within the Systems Frame: Reconciling the Differences." *Kairos: Slovenian Journal of Psychotherapy, 3*, 55–67.

Novo, P., Landin-Romero, R., Radua, J., Vicens, V., Fernandez, I., Garcia, F., Pomarol-Clotet., McKenna, P.J., Shapiro, F., & Amann, B.L. (2014). "Eye Movement Desensitization and Reprocessing Therapy in Subsyndromal Bipolar Patients with a History of Traumatic Events: A Randomized, Controlled Pilot-Study." *Psychiatry Research, 5*, 21–27.

Porges, S.W. (2011). *The Polyvagal Theory: Neurophysiological Foundations of Emotions, Attachment, Communication, and Self-Regulation.* New York: Norton.

Raboni, M.R., Tufik, S., & Suchecki, D. (2006). "Treatment of PTSD by Eye Movement Desensitization Reprocessing (EMDR) Improves Sleep Quality, Quality of Life, and Perception of Stress." *New York Academy of Sciences, 1071*, 508–513.

Schwartz, A. (2014). "Polyvagal Theory Helps Unlock Symptoms of PTSD." http://drarielleschwartz.com/polyvagal-theory-unlocks-symptoms-of-ptsd-dr-arielle-schwartz/#.WGxDgxsrl2w Accessed on January 6, 2017.

Shapiro, E., & Laub, B. (2009). "The Recent Traumatic Episode (R-TEP): An Integrative Protocol for Early EMDR Intervention (EEI)." emdrresearchfoundation.org/toolkit/rtep-luber-ch12.pdf Accessed on November 5, 2016.

Shapiro, E., & Laub, B. (2015). "Early EMDR Intervention Following a Community Incident: A Randomized Clinical Trial." *Journal of EMDR Practice and Research, 9*(1), 17–27.

Shapiro, F. (2001). *Eye Movement Desensitization and Reprocessing: Basic Principles, Protocols, and Procedures.* New York: The Guilford Press.

Shapiro, F. (Ed). (2002). *EMDR as an Integrative Psychotherapy Approach: Experts of Diverse Orientations Explore the Paradigm Prism.* Washington, DC: American Psychological Association.

Shapiro, F. (2007). "EMDR, Adaptive Information Processing, and Case Conceptualization." *Journal of EMDR Practice and Research, 1*(2), 68–87.

Shapiro, F. (2012). "Expert Answers on E.M.D.R." *New York Times Blog.* http://consults.blogs.nytimes.com/2012/03/16/expert-answers-on-e-m-d-r/ Accessed on December 12, 2016.

Silver, S.M., Rogers, S., Knipe, J., & Colelli, G. (2005). "EMDR Therapy following the 9/11 Terrorist Attacks: A Community-Based Intervention Project in New York City." *International Journal of Stress Management, 12*(1), 29–42.

Stickgold, R. (2002). "EMDR: A Putative Neurobiological Mechanism of Action." *Journal of Clinical Psychology, 58*(1), 61–75.

"Transcranial Magnetic Stimulation." (2015). *Mayo Clinic.* www.mayoclinic.org/tests-procedures/transcranial-magnetic-stimulation/home/ovc Accessed on December 5, 2016.

"Transcranial Magnetic Stimulation: Stimulation for the Treatment of Adults with PTSD, GAD, or Depression: A Review of Clinical Effectiveness and Guidelines." (2014). *Canadian Agency for Drugs and Technologies in Health.* www.ncbi.nlm.nih.gov/books/NBK254055/ Accessed on December 12, 2016.

van der Kolk, B.A. (2003). "The Neurobiology of Childhood Trauma and Abuse." *Child Adolescent Psychiatric Clinics of North America, 12*, 293–317.

van der Kolk, B.A. (2014). *The Body Keeps the Score: Brain, Mind, and Body in the Healing of Trauma.* New York: Viking.

Wylie, M.S. (2015). "The Limits of Talk: Bessel Van der Kolk Wants to Transform the Treatment of Trauma." *Psychotherapy Networker.* www.psychotherapynetworker.org/daily/article/485-the-limits-of-talk/ Accessed on December 16, 2016.

4 Enhancing the EMDR Protocol
An Integrated Approach

The integrated approach to EMDR that I hope to build in this chapter contains four components. First, I shall explore various intake, assessment, and diagnostic instruments that prepare the way for EMDR. Second, we will examine the role of attachment styles. An examination of the crucial Internal Family Systems (IFS) model will comprise the third stage of our investigation. Finally, a careful consideration of the major role played by mindfulness practices will round out our project. The result, I hope, will be an approach to EMDR that significantly enhances its effectiveness by drawing upon complementary tools in such a fashion that we can offer our clients a multifaceted, yet harmonious and organic, treatment experience that will have the greatest possible chance of success.

Intake, Screening, and Diagnostic Tools

The initial intake form that I utilize in my practice accesses a wide range of demographic information (e.g., name[s]; age; sex; marital status; education; occupation; current living situation; ethnicity; spirituality; worldviews; and financial levels). This intake form also assesses for the following: presenting complaint (e.g., symptoms, onset, duration, and severity); psychiatric history; family history; substance use history; trauma history; relationship history; social history; legal history; medical history; suicidality and homicidally; mental status; and treatment goals. When specifically assessing for trauma, I often initially, and periodically throughout the therapeutic process, administer the Beck's Depression Inventory (BDI), the Beck's Anxiety Inventory (BDA), and the Dissociative Experiences Scale (DES) since most trauma survivors suffer from anxiety and depression as well as from symptoms of dissociation.

In our 2011 article, "Healing from Trauma: Utilizing Effective Assessment Strategies to Develop Accessible and Inclusive Goals," my colleague Anibal Bernal Torres and I researched the efficacy of a multitude of assessments for PTSD/trauma, including: the PTSD Checklist-Civilian Version (PCL-C); the PTSD Checklist—Military Version (PCL-M); the Traumatic Life Events Questionnaire (TLEQ); the Clinician-Administered PTSD Scale for Adults (CAPS); the Life Events Checklist for DSM-V (LEC) (with CAPS); the Stressful Life Events Screening Questionnaire (SLESQ); the Traumatic History

Questionnaire (THQ); the Impact of Event Scale-Revised (IES-R); and The Harvard Traumatic Questionnaire (HTQ). My initial assessments for PTSD/trauma in clinical practice, however, prove to be the PTSD Checklist—Civilian Version (PCL-C), the PTSD Checklist—Military Version (PCL-M) and the PTSD Symptom Scale-Self-Report Version (PSS-SR-17) due to their validity, good temporal stability, internal consistency, test-retest reliability, and convergent reliability. I accompany them with a thorough clinical interview.

In their 2010 article "The Diagnostic Accuracy of the PTSD Checklist: A Critical Review," Scott D. McDonald and Patrick S. Calhoun provide additional support: "The PCL is the most commonly used PTSD self-report questionnaire, and it has been used extensively as a PTSD screening test, a diagnostic tool and an estimator of PTSD prevalence" (p. 85). As McDonald and Calhoun continue,

> The PCL has several strengths including favorable diagnostic accuracy in comparison with other shorter screens and its usefulness as a PTSD symptom tracking tool. When followed by a second-tier diagnostic test such as a standardized interview, the PCL can be a useful screening tool for clinical or research applications.
>
> (p. 985)

As even its supporters acknowledge, however, results of the PCL differ depending upon populations sampled and the research methods used. The PCL, like other self-report instruments, is not a stand-alone tool and cannot replace a thorough clinician interview (McDonald and Calhoun, 2010).

My use of the PCL is buttressed by other trauma assessments, including the Impact of Event Scale-Revised (IES-R) and followed by a standardized review such as the Clinician-Administered PTSD Scale (CAPS). The CAPS is a widely used semi-structured interview that assesses the features, frequency, and intensity of PTSD as well as tracking changes in diagnostic status and symptom severity over time. Another helpful tool in assessing trauma is the Harvard Traumatic Questionnaire (HTQ), which proves to be an open-ended, subjective, and cross-cultural instrument. When we add the History-taking and Assessment phases of EMDR, and the investigation of constraints in the six domains provided by the Metaframeworks perspective, (i.e., organization, sequences, mind, development, gender, and culture), discussed in detail in Chapter 5, I feel that the PCL is bolstered as a screening and diagnostic tool. However, the real quagmire in investigating the accuracy of screening for PTSD/trauma lies in the changes, as well as in what is missing, in the DSM-V's section on Trauma and Stress-Related Disorders. Many of the creators of PTSD assessment tools are already beginning the tedious and lengthy process of adapting these diagnostic tools to reflect the changes made in the DSM-V.

The genogram, an equally important assessment tool for individuals and family systems, warrants our attention here. The genogram provides an understanding of attachment issues, communication patterns, and relational conflicts that often arise from dysfunctional patterns such as fusion, emotional cutoffs, and triangles. Attachment, for example, refers to the connections established early on in one's life. If the child's needs are met, the attachment will be secure and enable the child to understand, and to appropriately control, thoughts and emotions. However, if their needs are not met, the attachment will be insecure, producing an inability to self-regulate and connect with others in a healthy way. This inability to self-regulate and connect with others often leads to *dissociation*—a state of being expressed in the development of separate personality parts, a negative sense of self, and memories that are not realized as an accurate narrative. Giving credit to the seminal work of Pierre Janet for the research evaluating the relationship between trauma and dissociation, van der Kolk reveals in his 2014 book *The Body Keeps the Score: Brain, Mind, and Body in the Healing of Trauma*, "Dissociation is the essence of trauma. The overwhelming experience is split off and fragmented, so that the emotions, sounds, images, thoughts, and physical sensations related to the trauma take on a life of their own" (p. 66). Thus the disruption of usually well-put-together functions of the conscious mind, memory and perception, must be addressed in trauma therapy, which deals with intense fragmentation, hypervigilance, irrational emotional overload, flashbacks, and negative somatic sensations (van der Kolk, 2014).

In his 2010 book *In an Unspoken Voice: How the Body Releases Trauma and Restores Goodness*, Peter A. Levine notes, "Trauma sufferers live in a world of chronic dissociation. This perpetual state of disembodiment keeps them disoriented and unable to engage in the here and now" (p. 355). In my experiences, my clients often attempt to dissociate from their past painful traumatic experiences in an effort to "block" that keeps them from integrating their past toxic experiences with their present toxic thoughts, feelings, and sensations. However, I have often discovered that when guided by mindfulness (discussed at length in the "Mindfulness" section in this chapter, pp. 75–81), my clients can move from being held captive by frozen fragments to experiencing a more gentle sense of wholeness.

In an 2010 article "Traumatic Stress, Affect Dysregulation, and Dysfunctional Avoidance: A Structural Equation Model," John Briere, Monica Hodges, and Natacha Godbout continue the thread:

> The finding that posttraumatic stress and affect regulation difficulties predicted unique variance in dysfunctional avoidance suggests multiple pathways to dysfunctional avoidance behaviors in interpersonal trauma survivors. Some individuals may respond to posttraumatic stress with dysfunctional avoidance, others may engage in dysfunctional avoidance primarily due to insufficient regulation capacity, and some may invoke dysfunctional avoidance in response to the additive combination of these variables.
>
> (pp. 772–773)

Most impressive for this author, whose concern is *integration*, is the ability of those working with Internal Family Systems Therapy (IFS) to make another seminal connection between trauma and dissociation. In her 2013 essay, "Integrating IFS with Phase-Oriented Treatment of Clients with Dissociative Disorder," for instance, Joanne H. Twombly notes:

From the perspective of IFS, people with complex PTSD and DDs have exiles who carry burdens of extreme emotion and beliefs, as well as firefighters and managers who are either rigidly controlling or easily overwhelmed. This complicates the inner family of a client with DD in a number of ways. Parts tend to be more dissociated and may seem to have no connections with each other; parts are often phobic of each other and do not want anyone, including the therapist, to know about them; and treatment is further complicated by the possibility of the inner family having layers of dissociated parts who reveal themselves only as progress is being made. As a result, the client who begins to function on a higher level can suddenly go into crisis.

(p. 72)

I will expand on the theoretical and practical IFS concepts later in this chapter as I continue to *enhance the EMDR protocol.*

Differentiation is another essential component understood when utilizing the genogram and Bowen Family Systems Therapy. It is the ability to balance a sense of togetherness and autonomy, and is crucial for the existence of a healthy and functional family system. When individuals in the family system are "fused," for example, the emphasis is placed on too much togetherness, while when the individuals within the family system have too little autonomy the result is an emotional cutoff. Fusion and cutoffs are extreme patterns that account for the reactivity we often see in those who suffer from trauma within the systems paradigm. In turn, triangles, which occur when two people in the system join against a third party in the system, increase the presence of dysfunctional patterns such as fusion and cutoffs.

The information culled from the genogram thus far provides EMDR clinicians with the ability to make accurate and necessary connections between the emotional reactivity in the client's present and their previously unprocessed traumatic memories. The theoretical framework in Bowen Family Systems Therapy exposes, for example, the presence of unresolved reactivity, internal and external polarities, differentiation of Self, recognition and healing of anxious attachment, the I-position, the function of triangles (created by friends, families, and even memories), *all of which enhances the efficacy of the Preparation phase in EMDR.* BFS Therapy and EMDR both posit that anxiety, frequently caused by toxic traumatic memories, threaten psychic equilibrium, and that we need to explore systems dynamics, rather than to explore symptomology alone.

In her 2007 article "Use of the Genogram with Families for Assessment and Treatment," Sylvia Shellenberger notes that "the genogram has been shown to be a powerful therapeutic tool for family systems therapy and as an adjunct to other forms of therapy such as EMDR" (p. 93). As Shellenberger continues,

> Genogram interviewing can be used to understand and to intervene with family systems of people of different ethnic and racial backgrounds, particular disorders and illnesses (e.g., substance abuse, Huntington's disease, HIV), social challenges (e.g., poverty, marginalization) and life crises (e.g.,

war, hurricanes). Through the genogram, EMDR targets may be identified and family system dynamics revealed.

(p. 93)

To put it quite simply, this author recognizes the importance of the concept that one's perceptions of the present are linked to the networks of unprocessed memories informed by earlier dysfunctional beliefs and relational communication patterns, emotions, and sensations perpetuated by multi-generations. Thus, successfully integrating two "seemingly" different theoretical and practical modalities, Bowen Family Systems Therapy and EMDR, into an adaptive resolution offers another comprehensive approach for healing a **world of trauma**.

In addition, the all-important use of the genogram in the Preparation stage of the EMDR protocol is crucial in our understanding of what takes place in the "meaning-making" of those suffering from trauma. A comprehensive and powerful joining tool, the genogram allows clinicians to collect and map complex family history and structure, mental health diagnoses, epigenetics, traumas, medical problems, and inter-relational patterns across multiple and diverse ethnic, racial, and cultural generations in a rapid and easily interpreted and structured format.

Furthermore, in obtaining such information, the genogram allows the EMDR clinician to help clients and their families comprehend that their past and the resulting learned patterns are contributing to their present struggles. From my perspective, this newly acquired wisdom helps those suffering from trauma to understand reactivity, to help them to break the negative cycle of repeating dysfunctional patterns, and to alter the negative cognitions (discussed in Chapter 3) that develop as a result of trauma: "I am not safe"; "I should have done something differently"; "I am not in control"; "I am not good enough"; just to name a few.

In her 2004 article "The Color Coded Timeline Trauma Genogram," Karin Jordan takes the genogram to a new level assessing multi-trauma events and primary and secondary trauma by implementing color coding to identify the type of trauma and letters to identify multi-trauma and primary and secondary trauma (Jordan, 2004). As Jordan notes, " The color-coded timeline trauma genogram (CCTTG) was developed in response to increasing abuse and violence in families, schools, businesses, and communities, as well as mass disasters (natural and human made) and the trauma of war" (p. 58). As Jordan continues,

> The CCTTG can serve as a systemic trauma assessment and intervention tool for systemic therapists. It can assist them in assessing the nature of the trauma, the affective, cognitive and behavioral responses to the trauma, the predisposing forces that increase trauma reactivity and possible trauma transmission of family patterns across generations.

(p. 59)

In her 2008 PhD dissertation, "The Family Genogram Interview: Reliability and Validity of a New Interview Protocol," Lisa F. Platt focuses on developing and testing the "psychometric properties" of the Family Genogram Interview (FGI), a 75-minute standardized interview protocol intended to expand on former structural and factual genogram formats by accessing family components such as "marital conflict," "emotional cutoff," "symptoms in a spouse," and "focus on a child." Platt posits that this method of inquiry helps clinicians assess for additional systemic stressors and patterns. Platt's study promises to make the genogram an even more effective assessment tool in working with individuals and families who suffer from trauma (see Platt, 2008). As such, I believe that integrating theoretical and practical modalities such as BFS Therapy, with an emphasis on the genogram, and EMDR have the potential to decrease the staggering statistics that suggest that we are all still living in a **world of trauma**.

In addition, there exists a category of assessments that are rarely utilized, particularly those assessments of "both complex trauma exposures" and "complex traumatic outcomes or adaptions," for children and adolescents suffering from complex trauma (addressed in Chapter 1). In their 2002 study "Complex Trauma in Children and Adolescents," the National Child Traumatic Stress Networks (NCTSN) explains, "In addition to assessing traumatic exposures, the clinicians must evaluate adaptations to complex trauma in seven domains: biology, attachment, affect regulation, dissociation, behavioral management, cognition and self-perception." The conductors of this study recognize the importance of initial evaluation, testing at periodic intervals to identify treatment progress as well as follow-up evaluation. The child/adolescent assessments include comprehensive evaluations such as "developmental history, family history, traumatic history for child and family, and coping skills," to name a few, as well as standardized measurements such as those mentioned in the introduction of this chapter (see www.NCTSNet.org).

Four particular assessment tools also deserve more thorough discussion here, namely, the Dissociative Experiences Scales (DES), the abbreviated version of The Mood Disorder Questionnaire (MDQ), the COPE Inventory, and The Adult Attachment Interview (AAI), given their recommendation as assessment tools in the EMDR protocol. The DES, for example, developed by Eve Bernstein Carlson and Frank W. Putnam, is a 28-item self-report whose screening format, which has shown to have validity and reliability, measures responses to statements such as, "Some people sometimes have the experience of feeling that other people, objects, and the world around them are not real," on a scale of 0% (never) to 100% (always).

The Mood Disorder Questionnaire instrument, a 13-question self-report assessment tool, was developed by a committee composed of "psychiatrists, researchers and consumer advocates" including: Robert M.A. Hirschfeld, Joseph F. Calabrese, Laurie Flynn, Paul E. Keck, Jr, Lydia Lewis, Robert M. Post, Gary S. Sachs, Robert L. Spitzer, Janet Williams, and John M. Zajecka to accurately assess bipolar disorder, which includes Bipolar I, Bipolar II, and Bipolar NOS. If left untreated, bipolar disorder can lead to a rate of suicidal completion of 19% according to a meta-analysis of ten studies, although rates vary considerably in the research (12%–60%). According to the team of professionals who developed this instrument, "Clinical trials have indicated that the MDQ has a high rate of accuracy; it is able to identify seven out of ten people who have bipolar disorder and screen out nine out of ten people who do not" (Chadis, n.d.). Studies have revealed that nearly 73% of individuals suffering from bipolar disorder have experienced being misdiagnosed at least once and not receiving an accurate diagnosis for more than 10 years from the onset presentation of their symptoms (Hirschfeld, 2002). Having read my Preface as well as the summary in Chapter 3 of a 2014 study supporting the efficacy of EMDR, "Eye Movement Desensitization and Reprocessing in in Subsyndromal Bipolar Patients with a History of Traumatic Events: A Randomized, Controlled Pilot-Study," I am sure my readers can recognize the necessity of utilizing this *integrated* assessment tool in enhancing the EMDR protocol.

The COPE Inventory is also a crucial assessment tool when treating psychological trauma since it is important to understand how clients cope when they experience stressful events. When a clinician takes on the role of treating psychological trauma, the challenges, however, move to a higher order. This questionnaire inquires about what clients do and feel when stressful experiences occur. As the creators of this inventory explain, "we feel that it is time to give more thought to what self-regulatory functions are implicit in people's coping effects. We think it should be useful to probe specific aspects of the coping process that may be important despite their not coming to mind most immediately as coping tactics" (Carver et al., 1989, p. 280).

The final assessment tool that I would highly suggest my readers consider utilizing in their practice given its importance in working with those suffering from psychological trauma is The Adult Attachment Interview (AAI). In his 2009 book *Mindsight: The New Science of Personal Transformation*, Daniel J. Siegel refers to the AAI as "the research instrument that measures how we have 'made sense' of our lives." As Siegel continues, "Answering this set of open-ended questions is like diving deeply into areas of untapped memory. When I was doing research with the AAI, many subjects told me that the interview was the most helpful therapy session they ever had" (pp. 173–174; see Siegel, 2009 for further discussion). This assessment tool, along with the three preceding ones, significantly aid the EMDR therapist in the formulation of the best-informed hypothesis.

Exploring Attachment Styles

When exploring attachment styles as they relate to trauma, we must consider, first and foremost, the trust experiences that individuals encounter with their caregivers such as neglect, emotional, physical, and sexual abuse, disconnects from attachment figures, and exposure to terrifying actions in attachment figures. Francine Schapiro's Adaptive Information Processing (AIP) Model (see Chapter 3) addresses the negative cognitions and beliefs that can develop and become contained in cognitive regions of the brain during childhood. In his 2014 essay, "Attachment, Anxiety, Internal Working Models," in his 2014 book *John Bowlby and Attachment Theory*, Jeremy Holmes defines attachment theory this way: "Attachment style refers to state and quality of an individual's attachments" (p. 53). Attachments can be secure or insecure. If they are secure (e.g., between 60% and 70% of the population), the individual trusts their caregivers, is comforted by them, and usually displays appropriate behaviors as well as experiences the sense of being safe in the world. If the attachments styles are insecure (i.e., avoidant, ambivalent, and disorganized), the presentation looks very different (Holmes, 2014).

In her 2006 article "Inducing Traumatic Attachment in Adults with a History of Child Abuse: Forensic Applications," Felicity de Zulueta codifies the development of three insecure attachments, namely, ambivalent (12% of the population), avoidant (20–25% of the population), and disorganized (15% of the population). The ambivalent group presents with anxious, clinging, and angry behavior in order to get the attention of their "inconsistent" and intrusive parents. The avoidant group is often emotionally dismissed by their parents and tends to avoid feeling vulnerable by acting unconcerned and refusing the need to be loved. This group can often become extremely fearful and depressed. The disorganized group often suffers from parents who are terrifying and abusive and experience terminal fear and are at a high risk for dissociation and emotional illness. Since traumatic experiences associated with attachment figures are stuck in neural networks that contain negative beliefs, images, and emotions, attachment figures are often primary triggers for maladaptive information. However, secure attachment can be achieved when trauma(s) are reprocessed, thus establishing a new adaptive perspective which then positively impacts future relationships (de Zulueta, 2006).

The confusion resulting from an individual's emotions not being addressed (e.g., fear, love, rejection, irritability, to mention a few) can often lead to pathology. One of the most complex populations to treat suffering from trauma and magnified by insecure attachment styles are those diagnosed with Borderline Personality Disorder, given the fact that their concurrent destructive behaviors also seriously impact their relationships with family members, romantic partners, and the mental health professionals who treat them. As Holmes remarks,

> The attachment perspective on BPD has several implications for treatment. The patient will lack a sense of a secure base. Extreme forms of avoidance and ambivalence are likely. The patient may resist any emotional involvement in therapy as a defense against the trauma that close relationships have entailed in the past, leaving the therapist with the uncomfortable feeling that he is inflicting therapy on an unwilling subject. Alternatively, the patient may cling to the therapy for dear life, leaving the therapists feeling stifled and guilty about leading comfortable non-work lives. There may be oscillations between these two positions: in one session the therapist feels she is really making progress, only to be faced at the next with an indifferent patient for whom the previous advance appeared to be an illusion.
>
> (p. 180)

Furthermore, Holmes considers the systemic implications of attachment styles when he reflects on Bowlby's theory by noting,

> Bowlby saw a person's attachment status as a fundamental determinant of their relationships. Whether smoothly functioning or problematic, core attachment patterns have a powerful influence on the way someone sees the world and their behavior. When there is a secure core state, a person feels good about themselves and their capacity to be effective and pursue their projects. When the core state is insecure, defensive strategies come into play.
> (p. 134)

As discussed in Chapter 1, individuals who present with trauma have difficulties regulating their emotions, and this is certainly compounded by insecure attachment styles. As Holmes goes on to explain, an insecurely attached person will likely have a compromised ability to read both their own emotions and the emotions of others. This difficulty in picking up on emotional signals can undo emotional regulation (Holmes, 2014).

In his 2010 book "*In an Unspoken Voice: How the Body Releases Trauma and Restores Goodness*, Peter A. Levine explores the neurobiological component to attachment issues. As Levine notes,

> Nervous systems are tuned to access potential risk in the environment—an unconscious evaluation process that Porges calls "neuroception." If one perceives the environment to be safe, one's social engagement system inhibits the more primitive limbic and brain stem structures that control flight or fright. After being moderately startled, you might, for example be calmed by another person—as when a mother says to her child. "It's ok; that was only the wind blowing." Generally, when threatened or upset, one first looks to others, wishing to engage their faces and voices and to communicate one's feelings to secure collective safety. These are called attachment behavior. Attachment is virtually the only defense young children have, as they cannot usually protect themselves by fighting or fleeing. Attachment for security is a general mammalian and primate survival strategy against predation.
> (pp. 98–99; see my discussion of Levine in Chapter 1)

An inherent need of individuals to attach is critical to all relationships, but particularly to those of an intimate nature (i.e., couples and partners). Individuals often choose a partner with characteristics absent from their family of origin in an effort to heal attachments' injuries/wounds. If a partner is unable to heal the attachment wounds and get past mistrust and insecurity, the relationship is often compromised. The good news is that attachment styles can change for both individuals and in their adult romantic partnerships, often with the help of EMDR. In his 2007 essay "Enhancing Attachments: Conjoint Couple Theory," Mark D. Moses explains,

Viewed from an EMDR Adaptive Informational Processing perspective, a couple's overreactions and overregulation (e.g., shutting down) in repetitive interactions are fueled by traumatic material encapsulated in the brain and triggered by one's partner. When incompletely processed and stored, small 't' (small traumas) attachment experiences become triggered, and distortions and other blocks can occur.

(Moses, 2007, p. 148)

However, if these targets are identified (see discussion of the genogram above), by both partners and empathetically witnessed and reprocessed (i.e., during the Desensitization phase of EMDR), I often find that the couple or intimate partners can process negative core beliefs and emotions altering their insecure attachment styles, interrupt negative family systems patterns, and improve communication, thus moving towards a more healthy relationship. When severe complex trauma (large "T") is present, however, it is considerably more difficult to resolve the couples' attachment styles. In these cases, additional resources and safety measures must be crafted into the Preparation phase of the EMDR protocol. The commitment level of each partner should also be assessed as well as the presence of hostile emotions and behaviors resulting from the presence of the following: domestic abuse; multiple and long-term physical, sexual, or emotional abuse; substance-related and addictive disorders; borderline personality disorder; dissociative disorders; and bipolar disorders (Moses, 2007).

When exploring attachment styles in children and adolescents suffering from complex posttraumatic trauma, it is crucial to place even more emphasis on exploring the early caregiving relationship since this is often a prediction of how this population perceives his or her self, and how they perceive themselves in relations to others. The child caregiver relationship is very often the source of the trauma. According to the NCTSN, "insecure attachment patterns have been consistently documented in over 80% of maltreated children" (www.NCTSNET.org).

Internal Family Systems (IFS)

Over a period of 30 years, Richard C. Schwartz developed the Internal Family Systems model (IFS), in part psychotherapeutic with an eye on neuroscience, in response to clients' descriptions of various parts within themselves. In 2001, he founded the Center for Self-Leadership (see www.selfleadership.org) which offers three levels of training and workshops in IFS for professionals and the general public, both in this country and abroad. The Internal Family Systems is in many ways comparable to the external family system in that it is made up of distinct personality parts engaged in complex sequences and interactions with one another. In his 2013 essay "An Introduction to IFS," Jack Engler explains "the mind is not a singular entity or self, but is multiple, composed of parts" (p. xviii). As Engler continues,

> This principle of multiplicity is at the core of the IFS model. Each of our parts, Dr. Schwartz found, has its own history, outlook and approach, its

own idiosyncratic beliefs, characteristic moods and feelings, and its own relationships with other parts. More important, each part has its own distinct role or function within the internal system.

(p. xviii)

There are three categories of IFS parts. The "managers," or protective parts, run our daily lives. They tend to be striving and controlling, obsessive and caretaking in an effort to achieve safety by keeping the second group, the "exiles" or "burdened" parts who carry emotional suffering and trauma and are isolated and frozen in the past, out of the picture. The "firefighters" are the third group, a protective part that desperately tries to "put out the pain" or intense emotion of the exiles when they are awakened by engaging in a number of risky behaviors including: substance abuse; sexual promiscuity; spending money; and self-destructive tendencies such as cutting and suicide to remove intense feelings. The "burdened" parts can manifest as feelings, thoughts, images, shapes, sensations, words, or physical symptoms. They can carry the essence of shame, fear, defectiveness, anger, guilt, self-criticism, and being invisible, among others.

One of the basic assumptions of the IFS model is that it *welcomes all parts* as long as they are not extreme. When any one part becomes extreme, it blends with another part or the "Self." Everyone has a "Self," our spiritual core which is open, nonjudgmental, and wise, and which should always be in a position of leadership in the internal family system. This differentiated-Self is described as having clarity (or wisdom), calmness, compassionate, confident, creativity, curiosity, courage, and connectedness. The goal of IFS therapy is to recognize the differences between the "Self" and the parts, to achieve balance among the parts, and to get the "Self" to lead. In order to achieve this end, it is necessary to decrease the extreme roles that the "managers," "exiles," and "firefighters" can, and often do, take on and un-blend these parts from each other and the "Self." The role of the IFS therapist is to patiently create an environment of safety, build resources, and demonstrate compassion and curiosity for all parts. The IFS therapist also gently helps clients access, and, in a sometimes playful manner, witness and un-blend extreme and polarized parts, removing the wounded beliefs and feelings and cognitions in a non-judgmental way, thus enabling memory reintegration. If the parts are left extreme and polarized, these parts can, literally, "squash the Self" (Sweezy and Ziskind, 2013).

In my clinical practice, I assess the protective parts first and demonstrate respect for their concerns and safety. I monitor resistance when they are extreme and help them to engage in a dialogue with other parts. When one part, namely a manager, is clearly too extreme, however, I might ask if she is willing to "step out of the room" so that some of the differentiated parts of the Self can dialogue with a terrified, unprotected, burdened exile part. As Engler summarizes, "It was the work of slowly un-blending from terrified parts, befriending and reaching out to frightened protectors, and being able to work with them all from Self, that enabled me to gradually find some balance and inner peace" (p. xxiii).

For this author, the IFS model offers a holistic, collaborative, and *integrated* approach much like the EMDR protocol as well as the larger purpose of my book. Understanding the relationship among clients' individual parts, for example, is crucial to strengthening the Preparation phase of the EMDR protocol which addresses safety, stabilization, and a more positive sense of Self.

Mindfulness

As Levine pithily addresses the importance of mindfulness in his 2010 book *In an Unspoken Voice: How the Body Releases Trauma and Restores Goodness*, "In a lifetime of working with traumatized individualizes, I have been struck by the intrinsic and wedded relationship between trauma and spirituality" (p. 347), with "spirituality" serving as a general category embracing the sort of self-cultivation that is mindfulness.

According to Levine, "Once people learn to access this rhythmic flow within, 'infinite' emotional pain begins to feel manageable and finite. This allows their attitude to shift from dread and helplessness to curiosity and exploration" (p. 351). This is in essence self-regulation, the ability to sit with the painful traumatic physical and emotional sensations and cope with environmental difficulties.

Mindfulness is an essential component of spirituality. In his 2013 essay, "Mindfulness: What Is It? What Does It Matter?" Christopher Germer explains: "The term mindfulness is an English translation of the *Pali* word *Sati*. Pali was the language of Buddhist psychology 2,500 years ago, and mindfulness is the core teaching of this tradition. *Sati* connotes *awareness, attention, and remembering*" (p. 5). Mindfulness stems from the concepts arising from Buddhist psychology's dedication to alleviating suffering. The "Buddha," a person who is awake, recognized that the human condition involves suffering and that suffering can be removed by insight and diligent effort.

Mindfulness does not conflict with any non-Buddhist religious beliefs or traditions since it is based on philosophy, not upon theology or religious doctrine. Buddhist psychology is an all-encompassing program that trains the mind and "cultivates happiness" (Germer, 2013). There are both similarities and differences between the Buddhist tradition of mindfulness and Western psychotherapy's adaptation of it. While highly theoretical analyses of the relationship between Buddhism and Western thought are beyond the purview of this book, they are elegantly addressed in *Mindfulness and Psychotherapy* (Germer, 2013) by a host of scholars in the field.

An equally technical matter, namely, the neurobiological components of mindfulness, is covered in the same publication. The authors, for example, bring to our attention the scientific community's recent focus on neuroplasticity. Neuroplasticity posits that changes in our brain structure are, in fact, possible and that connections in the brain change in response to our experiences.

These changes are now believed by many in the scientific community to impact a shift in behaviors including coping with difficult situations, developing better attention and memory skills, and enhancing compassion. This suggests that mindfulness, paying attention to the present moment with greater awareness, can also utilize neuroplasticity. In addition, mindfulness meditation coupled with the research on neuroplasticity suggests that activation in the amygdala, a part of the brain powerfully engaged in trauma, can be decreased. For example, Richard J. Davidson and Antoine Lutz in their 2007 article "Buddha's Brain: Neuroplasticity and Meditation" point out that "this finding may support the idea that advanced levels of concentration [mindfulness] are associated with a significant decrease in emotionally reactive behaviors that are incompatible with stability of concentration" (p. 173). In essence, getting some distance from the content of trauma, observing the effect the trauma is having on them and separating from it, the practice of mindfulness reminds those suffering from trauma that according to the concept of neuroplasticity, the brain can actually be rewired. In turn, the awareness practiced as part of the EMDR protocol could be further enhanced by those suffering from trauma by practicing mindfulness.

In my opinion, the more basic similarities between Buddhist psychology/ mindfulness and our Western psychotherapeutic adoption and adaptation of mindfulness are potent and clearly translate into the awareness that our way of living is fluid and constantly changing. This fusion of perspectives helps us in remembering what is and what is not, as well as what is correct and what incorrect. It makes us aware of the need to leave our own agendas behind and to see things in their natural state, what Buddhists would call their simple "suchness." This partnership between East and West allows us to experience "mind" in its purest, most organic form and to notice the present moment.

Mindfulness also cultivates an active curiosity about what is occurring in the present moment, free of judgment or expectation. Jon Kabat-Zinn is a pioneer who created the Center for Mindfulness at the University of Massachusetts Medical School in 1979 to treat many chronic conditions, and who by 2012 had created over 700 MBSR (Mindfulness Based Symptom Reduction) programs worldwide (Germer, 2013). As Kabat-Zinn explains in his book *Wherever You Go, There You Are: Meditation in Everyday Life* (2005), "Mindfulness means paying attention in a particular way: on purpose, in the present moment, and nonjudgmentally. This kind of attention nurtures greater awareness, clarity, and acceptance of present-moment reality" (p. 4).

Kabat-Zinn's insights imply that mindfulness is a curiosity and openness, simply observing what is happening without bias, with a stillness that receives, observes, and describes. Mindfulness, thus, becomes a vehicle of insight, an opportunity to be free from clinging to judgment, to reorganize deep thoughts and welcome them, and to tolerate and accept them along with the diverse body sensations and emotional patterns that present in all those who suffer from trauma (Kabat-Zinn, 2005).

Stephen Porges explores the benefits of cultivating mindfulness with self-regulation in those who suffer from trauma in his 2010 book *The Polyvagal Theory*:

> Victims of abuse have state regulation difficulties with a bias toward behavioral states that are self-protective. This potential vulnerability to become defensive may result in difficulties in feeling safe with others and in developing trusting social relationships. A self-awareness of difficulties in regulating state, especially staying calm in the presence of others, may lead individuals to seek alternative strategies, such as yoga. Yoga exercises may help reduce symptoms of depression and anxiety, increase a sense of self-efficacy, and improve regulation of the autonomic nervous system. Thus individuals who practice yoga may be exercising their autonomic nervous system in an attempt to normalize an abuse-related damage to their ability to self-regulate.
>
> (p. 240)

As such, mindfulness as well as yoga enhance self-regulation and subsequently can be an effective antidote to psychological distress, which makes it a powerful resource for treating PTSD.

The mind becomes corrupted when negative and fearful emotions enter our unconscious or conscious states. As Germer notes, "Mindfulness is a skill that allows us to be less reactive to what is happening in the moment. It is a way of relating to all experience—positive, negative, and neutral—such that our overall suffering diminishes and our sense of well-being increases" (p. 4). In essence, this implies that by noticing the obvious—our breathing, our emotions, and our sensations—while carrying out our everyday tasks in a mindful way and from a non-judgmental stance, we can free ourselves from the constraints of "permanence," which Buddhists regard as an illusion that keeps us stuck in our suffering.

Mindfulness can be practiced in a formal or informal way but it must be practiced consistently with effort and discipline and with the intent of not resisting and of "letting go" (Germer, 2013).

In his 2006 essay "An Interpersonal Neurobiology Approach to Psychotherapy," Daniel J. Siegel brings the practice of mindfulness into the systemic frame. As Siegel recognizes, "Our brains are profoundly social. The structure of our neural architecture reveals that we need connections to other people to feel in balance and to develop well" (p. 254). Ronald Siegel expands the power of mindfulness in the systemic frame when he further notes,

> Mindfulness can help us get along with one another better. It helps us to see the other person more clearly and not believe so much in our judgements. So, we don't get caught as much in condemning the other person who has upset us today. It also helps us to not take things so personally. So, we can realize that much of the time, the other person's behavior, even

if it's disturbing to us, isn't really about us. Rather, it reflects their own struggles at the moment.

(p. 6)

Memories of trauma and the resulting negative emotions (grief, sadness, woundedness, anger, and fear, for instance), sensations, and cognitions when left untreated can become encoded in the brain and lead to PTSD and many other mental health diagnoses including, but not limited to, depression, anxiety, substance abuse, dissociation, and personality disorders. While there are few evidence-based studies of mindfulness interventions alone for those who suffer from trauma/PTSD and the resulting negative cognitions and avoidance, mindfulness can aid the EMDR protocol since part of the healing process is reintegrating one's physical and spiritual self along with the traumatic imprint. I have found that if you attend to the client's mind, you have also to address their somatic and spiritual self.

Mindfulness, a powerful tool in and of itself for gaining awareness and getting unstuck, works in tandem with EMDR's phase of Preparation/stabilization. Similarly, they are both a valuable resource for promoting safety, tolerating emotions, and self-regulating (confidence in experiencing unpleasant experiences) and allowing those suffering from trauma to self-soothe. They can decrease rumination, help the client recognize the concept of impermanence, as well as allowing her or him to become comfortable within this paradigm. In addition, this integration of paradigms helps the client stay safe, increases his self-confidence, and promotes reintegration of her memory and somatic experiences. The Adaptive Information Processing (AIP) model of EMDR is promoted by the practice of mindfulness by utilizing the client's own ability to heal and receive more positive cognitions more readily (see Chapter 3). As discussed in Chapter 3, resource development is a crucial component in integrating mindfulness and EMDR. This means identifying the presenting issue, as well as the qualities, capacities, skills, strengths, and resources already in place for these clients, in addition to those resources they might envision in the future, all of which enable a better sense of control and self-efficacy among those who suffer from trauma.

Mindfulness also enhances EMDR treatment by introducing the client's awareness of the flow of experience, strengthening her/his ability to create a vivid "safe place," a place that is comfortable, secure, peaceful, and personal in which they can focus on the image/target, feel the emotions that arise and sustain comfort in the face of fear and pain, and identify and tolerate all the parts of the Self and the accompanying somatic responses. As discussed in Chapter 3, EMDR therapists use bilateral stimulation to solidify these images and sensations by locating a "cue" word that allows the client to access their safe place quickly both during and between sessions, promoting an ability to relax during stressful moments. Trust, however, is one of the most important parts to merging mindfulness with EMDR's safety phase. If our clients do not trust our competence in mindfulness and in EMDR, our ability to be compassionate and empathize with suffering will be seriously compromised.

In mindfulness we are also suggesting that clients notice negative images, emotions, and sensations and attain the ability to simply flow through the experience by recognizing that these images, thoughts, emotions, and sensations are, in fact, impermanent, increasing the client's ability to cope effectively with disturbance and differentiating their core "Self" from these thoughts, emotions, and sensations. Using the breath to cultivate mindfulness is a potent tool to counter negative emotions, feelings, and sensations. By simply recognizing the breath coming in and out of one's body, there is implied focus on staying in the moment. Simple as this recognition can be, if impatience, blaming, or lack of motivation is present, all will be lost. How, then, do we convince those invested in these concepts to change? I often use the example of the Dalai Lama, who when questioned about the Chinese genocide toward his fellow Tibetans and his lack of anger, responded, "They have taken everything from us, should I let them take my mind as well?" This implies that although feelings of anger can occur for anyone (including our) patients, when they arise, mindfulness can be the "cure." There are a number of mindfulness exercises that I will offer in the appendices of this volume that have been developed by others that lend practical support to the theoretical framework of how mindfulness enhances the EMDR protocol.

In the end, then, in order to stay focused in the present in a nonjudgmental way, we need to cultivate attention to our feelings, emotions, and sensations/wisdom, and to recognize that suffering will always exist, but that by being present we develop an awareness that leads to compassion, a word that derives from the Latin roots *pati* (to suffer) and *con* (with), and when acquired, leads to our capacity for suffering with another person. Here we encounter the crucial interpersonal, dialogical component of mindfulness. As Janet L. Surry and Gregory Kramer recognize in their insightful 2013 essay "Relational Mindfulness,"

> We are wired for relationships, and our survival depends on relationships to live. We must rely on others for safety, comfort, and love as children and throughout our lives. We form bonds of attachment that impact all future relationships, and we're shaped not only by our own suffering as human beings, but also vicariously by the suffering of others.
>
> (p. 106)

In his 2006 essay already mentioned, Daniel J. Siegel posits some insightful connections between neurobiology and psychotherapy regarding relational and therapeutic mindfulness that carry "profound implications." "Mediated via the insula," notes Siegel, "perceptions of another's affective expressions may alter our own somatic and limbic states and then be examined through a prefrontal process of interoception, interpretation, and attribution to another's states" (p. 254). In what Siegel refers to as a "Mirror

Neuron-Mindfulness Hypothesis," for example, he explains, "Discovered in the mid-nineteen nineties, the mirror neuron system reveals how the brain is capable of integrating perceptual learning with motor action to create internal representations of intentional states in others" (p. 254). As Siegel continues, "For example, the mirror neuron system is thought to be an essential aspect of the neural basis for empathy. By perceiving the expressions of another person, the brain is able to create an internal state that is thought to 'resonate' with that of the other" (p. 254). "Being open to our own bodily states as therapists," reveals Siegel, "is a crucial step in establishing the interpersonal attunement and understanding that is at the heart of interpersonal integration" (p. 259).

In his 2010 book, *The Mindful Therapist: A Clinician's Guide to Mindsight and Neural Integration*, Siegel elaborates on what mindfulness signifies for contemporary clinicians and their relationship to their clients. He furthers our grasp of the complexity of mindfulness, describing Presence, Attunement, and Resonance, in turn. He describes Presence as "the way in which we are grounded in ourselves, open to others, and participate fully in the life of the mind are important aspects of our presence at the heart of relationships that help others grow" (p. xx). Attunement is defined in this way by Siegel:

> As signals are sent from one person to the other, we have the opportunity to tune in to those incoming streams of information and attend fully to what is being sent rather than becoming swayed by our own preconceived ideas or perceptual biases. When we attune to others—even in the urgency of an emergency visit—we offer a crucial open mind to listen deeply to what the patient needs to let us know.
>
> (p. xx).

And "With Resonance," concludes Siegel, "we come to 'feel felt' by the other. The joining has profound transformative effects on both people. This experience of connection brings with it a feeling of security, of being seen, and of feeling safe" (p. xx). This suggests to me that our role as *mindful* therapists is to have Presence, to stay Attuned, and to be open to Resonance with our clients and to encourage them to form such connections with the "other."

While there are many mindfulness exercises implemented in my sessions to manage anxiety, decrease rumination, change toxic emotions and feelings, and prepare clients for facing toxic memories such as the one in Appendix 6, one in particular, "Feeding Your Demons," (see Appendix 7), developed by Lama Tsultrim Allione (2016), often produces an epiphany among my clients. In the eleventh-century, the Tibetan female Buddhist master named Machig Labdron provided a practice for dealing with our inner demons in a productive fashion. Taking off from this classic technique, contemporary mindfulness practitioner and teacher Lama Tsultrim Allione has helpfully provided an exercise for "feeding our demons"—those factors in our life that enervate us—rather than simply opposing them. She takes us through five imaginative steps, focusing on personifying our personal demons and, ultimately, reintegrating their energy into a holistic sense of self such that one can "rest in awareness" (Allione, 2016, pp. 33–35). I also encourage interested readers to consider Allione's 2008 book *Feeding Your Demons: Ancient Wisdom for Resolving Inner Conflict* for a more thorough and insightful understanding of the Chod lineage of Machig Labdron that Allione has practiced since 1973 as well as her website, taramandala.org.

Summary

The human brain, and the mind to which it gives rise, is the most complex entity that we have yet encountered in the universe. Two important conclusions follow from this fact. First, we should not be surprised that the dysfunctions to which the human mind is subject are themselves often complex. The second conclusion is closely related: it makes little sense to suppose that we can effectively treat mind maladies with single instruments. EMDR is already a wonderfully comprehensive and artfully developed treatment modality, but it can potentially be made even more effective by joining it with complementary techniques. By doing so, we can offer our clients the kind of highly articulated healing programs that honor the multidimensional and sometimes tangled nature of the human mind.

References

Allione, L.T. (2008). *Feeding Your Demons: Ancient Wisdom for Resolving Inner Conflict*. New York: Little, Brown and Company.

Allione, L.T. (2016). "Feeding Your Demons." *Lion's Roar*, 1 (4), 33–35.

Briere, J., Hodges, M., & Godbout, N. (2010). "Traumatic Stress, Affect Regulation, and Dysfunctional Avoidance: A Structural Equation Model." *Journal of Traumatic Stress*, 23 (6), 767–774.

Carver, C.S., Scheier, M.F., & Weintraub, J.K. (1989). "Assessing Coping Strategies: A Theoretically Based Approach." *Journal of Personality and Social Psychology*, 56, 267–283.

Chadis. (n.d.). "Mood Disorder Questionnaire (MDQ)." www.chadis.com/site/content/mood-disorder-questionnaire-mdq Accessed September 16, 2016.

Davidson, R.J., & Lutz, A. (2007). "Buddha's Brain: Neuroplasticity and Meditation." *Ieee Signal Processing Magazine*, 176, September, 171–174.

de Zulueta, F. (2006). "Introducing Traumatic Attachment in Adults with a History of Child Abuse: Forensic Applications." *British Journal of Forensic Practice*, 8 (3), 4–15.

Engler, J. (2013). "An Introduction to IFS." *IFS Internal Family Systems Therapy: New Dimensions* (pp. xvii–xxvii). New York: Routledge: Taylor & Francis Group.

Germer, C.K. (2013). "Mindfulness: What Is It? What Does It Matter?" *Mindfulness and Psychotherapy* (pp. 3–35). Ed. Christopher K. Germer, Rondal D. Siegel, Paul R. Fulton. New York: Guilford Press.

Hirschfeld, R. (2002). "The Mood Disorder Questionnaire: A Simple, Patient-Related Screening Instrument for Bipolar Disorder." *Prime Care Companion Journal of Clinical Psychiatry*, 4 (1), 9–11.

Holmes, J. (2014). *John Bowlby and Attachment Theory* (2nd ed.). New York: Routledge: Taylor & Francis Group.

Jordan, K. (2004). "The Color Coded Timeline Trauma Diagram." *Brief Treatment Crises, 4*(1), 57–70.

Kabat-Zinn, J. (2005). *Wherever You Go, There You Are: Meditation in Everyday Life.* New York: Hachette Books.

Levine, P.A. (2010). *In an Unspoken Voice: How the Body Releases Trauma and Restores Goodness.* Berkeley, CA: North Atlantic Books.

McDonald, S.D., & Calhoun, P.S. (2010). "The Diagnostic Accuracy of the PTSD Checklist: A Critical Review." *Clinical Psychological Review, 30,* 976–987.

Mille, D., & Torres, B.A. (2011). "Healing from Trauma: Utilizing Effective Assessment Strategies to Develop Accessible and Inclusive Goals." *Kairos: Slovenian Journal of Psychotherapy,* 5, 25–39.

Moses, M.D. (2007). "Enhancing Attachments: Conjoint Couple Therapy." In F. Shapiro, F.W. Kaslow, & L. Maxfield, eds., *Handbook of EMDR and Family Therapy Processes* (pp. 146–168). Hoboken, NJ: John Wiley & Sons.

National Child Traumatic Stress Networks (NCTSN). (2002). "Complex Trauma in Children and Adolescents." www.NCTSNet.org Accessed on November 29, 2016.

Platt, L. (2008). *The Family Genogram Interview: Reliability and Validity of a New Interview Protocol.* Ph.D. Dissertation from Penn State University, Graduate School of Education.

Porges, S.W. (2010). *The Polyvagal Theory: Neurophysiological Foundations of Emotions, Attachment, Communication, and Self-Regulation.* Berkeley, CA: North Atlantic Books.

Shapiro, F., Kaslow, F.W., & Maxfield, L. (Eds). (2007). *EMDR and Family Therapy Processes.* Hoboken, New Jersey: John Wiley & Sons.

Shellenberger, S. (2007). "Use of the Genogram with Families for Assessment and Treatment." *Handbook of EMDR and Family Therapy Processes* (pp.76–94). Ed. Francine Shapiro, Florence W. Kaslow, and Louise Maxfield. Hoboken, NJ: John Wiley and Sons.

Siegel, D.J. (2006). "An Interpersonal Neurobiology Approach to Psychotherapy." *Psychiatric Annals, 36* (4), 248–256.

Siegel, D.J. (2009). *Mindsight: The New Science of Personal Transformation.* New York: Penguin Random House.

Siegel, D.J. (2010). *The Mindful Therapist: A Clinician's Guide to Mindsight and Neural Integration.* New York and London: W.W. Norton and Company.

Siegel, R.D. (2014). *The Science of Mindfulness: a Researched-Based Path to Well Being.* Chantilly, VA: The Teaching Company.

Surrey, J.L., & Kramer, G. (2013). "Relational Mindfulness." In C.K. Gerner, R.D. Siegel, & P.R. Fulton (Eds.), *Mindfulness and Psychotherapy.* (pp. 94–111). New York: The Guilford Press.

Sweezy, M., & Ziskind, E.L. (Eds). (2013). *Internal Family Systems Therapy.* New York and London: Routledge and Taylor and Francis Group.

Twombly, J.H. (2013). "Integrating IFS with Phase-Oriented Treatment of Clients with Dissociative Disorder." *Internal Family Systems Therapy: New Dimensions* (pp. 72–89). New York: Routledge: Taylor and Francis Group.

van der Kolk, B. (2014). *The Body Keeps the Score: Brain, Mind, and Body in the Healing of Trauma.* New York: Viking.

5 Utilizing the Metaframeworks Perspective to Enhance the Effectiveness of EMDR in Clinical Practice

This chapter continues the integrated thread of the systemic mindful paradigm offered by Siegel earlier through a dual exploration. I will first consider the general extant literature in exploring utilizing EMDR within the family systems therapy modality as well as the studies integrating the use of EMDR with specific family therapy models within the couple subsystem. My subsequent discussions will focus on enhancing the effectiveness of the neurobiological EMDR protocol by integrating it with one particular, and carefully crafted, family systems therapy model, namely the Metaframeworks perspective, an integration which, as far as I am aware, has never been researched or utilized from a clinical perspective. And I will explore how I use this approach with internal and external family systems in my practice.

The language provided for us by the Internal Family Systems (IFS) model codifies what I mean by the internal and external family systems and how this relates to my integrated and systemic approach in treating trauma (see previous chapter). In her 2013 essay "Self in Relationship: An Introduction to IFS Couple Therapy," Toni Herbine-Blank's goal as a couples therapist is to enable loving relationships both between the partners and among the parts constituting their internal, individual systems. As Herbine-Blank elucidates it,

> Internal Family Systems (IFS) invites people first to learn how to be in a loving relationship with themselves and, from that state, to attempt a heartfelt connection with their intimate partner. We offer the concepts of parts and Self to help couples reframe their bitter struggles and understand relationships differently.
> (Sweezy and Ziskind, 2013, p. 55)

As Herbine-Blank succinctly clarifies,

> We work with the internal system much as we would work with the external system, learning about the roles and protective functions of the parts, supporting the development of relationships between parts, and between parts and Self, and then helping our clients to access vulnerable young parts who carry the burdens of relational trauma. As the internal system

shifts we can usually observe positive effects on external relationships as well. In brief we see the external mirroring the internal. We always keep in mind that the painful polarizations, fears, conflict, rage and withdrawal that we see between partners are also occurring internally between the parts of each client.

(p. 58)

I am certain that at this point my readers are also well acquainted with how the horrific and negative effects of trauma can wreak havoc on the individual and those around them. However, in his 2014 book *The Body Keeps the Score: Brain, Mind and Body in the Healing of Trauma*, van der Kolk reminds us, "Trauma affects not only those who are directly exposed to it, but also those around them" (p. 1).

While they are not engaging in the use of EMDR, Susan M. Johnson and Lyn Williams-Keeler appear to be among the first authors who carefully consider healing couples with trauma where one or both of the partners have experienced significant trauma. The authors use a Family Systems Therapy (FST) modality, namely Emotionally Focused Therapy (EFT), when treating couples with trauma. In their 1998 study, "Creating Healing Relationships for Couples Dealing With Trauma: The Use of Emotionally Focused Marital Therapy," the authors explain: "EFT, in this context of trauma, incorporates the nine steps of conventional EFT and also encompasses the three stages of the 'constructivist' self-development theory of trauma treatment" (p. 25). As Johnson et al. defines it, "EFT is a short term (12–20 sessions) approach to marital therapy which focuses on reprocessing the emotional responses that organize attachment behaviors." As Johnson et al. continue,

> The EFT therapist works on both intrapsychic and interpersonal levels. On the intrapsychic level the therapist uses experiential techniques such as empathetic reflection and validation, and expands emotional experience by heightening and conjecture. On the inter-personal/systemic level, the therapist reflects and reframes the patterns and cycles in the interaction and directly choreographs new interactions and specific change events.
> (Johnson and Williams-Keeler, 1998, p. 29)

"The EFT therapist," continue Johnson and Williams-Keeler, "attempts to take clients to the leading edge of their experience as it occurs in the session and helps them to formulate the experience in new ways that evoke new responses both to and from their partner" (p. 29).

The nine steps of conventional therapy correspond with the three stages of their trauma treatment, and the EFT must attend to this process. For example, after the initial assessment phase, the stabilization (steps 1–4 of EFT) is attempted (i.e., identifying the negative interactions connected with trauma that the partners become aware of how each has suffered in the process ow the emotional aspects of their relationship can precipitate traumatic triggers). Establishing reflection, validation, and safety by the therapist are especially critical at this stage. The next phase, building self and interactive capacities (Steps 5–7 of EFT), is centered around helping couples interact in more nurturing ways (i.e., connection and trust) around the processing of the negative effects that occur when reprocessing trauma (i.e., attachment insecurity, fear, self-loathing, hurt, grief, betrayal, among others). In the integration phase (Steps 8–9 of EFT), the client is expected to experience a new sense of self built around the trust of their partner so that they can manage ongoing trauma issues (Johnson and Williams-Keeler, 1998).

While it is apparent from Johnson's and Williams-Keeler's study that EFT offers relief to couples suffering from some traumas due to attachment issues, or when the trauma seriously impacts their ability to support positive and close relationships, there appears to be something missing. By contrast, EMDR provides a neurobiological basis—its Adaptive Information Processing (AIP) approach, the three-pronged approach, and Shapiro's evidence-based research protocol to reprocess toxic memories (see Chapter 3)—that EFT does not include. Furthermore, the latter is not recommended for many psychological traumas and especially not for complex psychological trauma (Johnson and Williams-Keeler, 1998). Nonetheless, the qualified affirmations of the model above take me back to Siegel's concept of resonance when he notes, "Understanding others is extremely important: the interest in and intention to grasp another's point of view is a critical element in healing relationships" (Siegel, 2010, p. 55).

In her Preface in the 2007 book *The Handbook of EMDR and Family Therapy Processes*, Shapiro recognizes the benefits of integrating EMDR with Family Systems Therapy (FST). As she explains, "When EMDR has prepared the client to relate to family members without the burden of reactive emotional baggage, FST can help teach family members how to interact with each other more positively and provide new models for healthy interpersonal communication" (p. xxii). "In turn," as Shapiro continues, "EMDR processing can help accelerate the learning process by incorporating templates for positive future functioning" (p. xxii). However, in their 2007 essay "The Integration of EMDR and Family Systems Therapies," Louise Maxfield, Florence W. Kaslow, and Francine Shapiro also recognize that "the approaches of EMDR and FST are generally very different. They differ in theory, identification of the patient, focus, temporal view, and desired outcomes" (p. 407).

The goals of EMDR and FST are dissimilar since FST is based on the assumption of circular causality, where one person's actions are viewed as influencing another's in any system, and the EMDR protocol is a neurobiological protocol used to reprocess an individual's traumatic experiences. As Shapiro makes clear, EMDR is intended to reprocess troubling memories, thus eliminating their unwanted emotional affects and reworking trauma-related thinking (see Chapter 3). "In FST," explain Maxfield et al., "assessment and intervention are focused on issues related to family structure, dynamic patterns of interaction, boundaries, roles, rules, myths, expectations and communications. The primary purposes of treatment are to change the family's dysfunctional interactional patterns and expectations" (p. 409).

On the other hand, most of us would agree with Shapiro's belief that the "primary goal is to address the entire clinical picture to bring about the most comprehensive treatment effects" (quoted in Maxfield et al., 2007, p. 407). In the end, while the goals of EMDR and FST are variant, we must, as these authors above suggest, utilize an integrated approach in healing trauma.

Anita Bardin also supports the importance of enhancing EMDR with FST in her 2004 article "EMDR within a Family Systems Perspective." As Bardin explains, "The Trauma Unit of the Shiluv Institute for Family and Couple Therapy that I work with integrates its individual experiences treating trauma victims, especially through EMDR, with systemic and contextual family therapy. We see the victim, his traumatic experience, and his symptomatic behaviors as being part of, and affecting, his family system" (p. 49). In her study, Bardin presents the case of a nine-year old boy who was stabbed and explores the dynamic between the boy and four other family members consisting of the boy's mother and father, his 17-year older brother, who was also attacked, and his 14-year old brother, all of whose intensive feelings could have undermined EMDR if they had not been included in the therapeutic process (Bardin, 2004).

Furthermore, as discussed in my previous chapter, utilizing a diverse set of intake, screening, and diagnostic tools; assessing insecure attachment styles, injuries, and attachment issues; as well as assessing for dissociation and coping skills provides significant and necessary preparatory information for the therapist before embarking on the EMDR journey. As my readers have witnessed, for example, looking through the lens of Shapiro's AIP model, a couple's reactivity is often informed by earlier individual toxic traumatic memories which keep them *lost in translation*. This has almost always proved to be the case in my clinical practice with couples.

Previous insightful attempts have been made to integrate EMDR into couples' therapy. Mark D. Moses, for example, thoughtfully considers this integration in his 2007 contribution "Enhancing Attachments: Conjoint Couple Therapy." In his clearly articulated research and practical application, Moses realizes the importance of first working through attachment issues with family therapy models such as Conjoint Family Therapy, a combination of Emotionally Focused Therapy (EFT), psychodynamic therapy (Objective Relations), and Social Construction (Narrative Therapy) in an effort for clients to disclose their stressful narratives, practice more effective systemic skills, and obtain a more empathetic therapeutic environment. Moses also utilizes the EMDR protocol to re-process the remaining attachment issues, always a critical component in my own clinical work. I recommend that my readers refer to Moses's essay, as well as to Debra Wesselmann's equally informative 2007 essay, "Treating Attachment Issues through EMDR and a Family Systems Approach," in the same publication, which takes the methodology of processing remaining attachment issues through Shapiro's eight-phase trauma protocol via the lens of a well-crafted case study. I also applaud these authors for recognizing the circumstances when couple therapy might not be warranted when engaging in the EMDR protocol such as in the presence of severe and complex trauma, and when resistance, aggression, and emotional intensity are "off the charts." To this list, based on my clinical guidelines, I would also avoid implementing the EMDR protocol in cases when severe dissociation, extreme active substance, or domestic abuse, and severe co-morbid mental health diagnoses present within the couple subsystem. In the end, I support Moses' awareness that

> Each partner brings strengths and issues to the relationship. The etiologies of many attachment issues are found in small 't' trauma experiences, resulting in attachment limitations, such as bonds that are blocked by impasses. In contrast, large 'T' traumas, that is, those related to life-threatening events, such as assault, abuse, and other serious trauma, require special assessments and cautions to determine if conjoint EMDR is indicated or contraindicated.
>
> (p. 162)

Another 2002 essay, "EMDR in Conjunction with Family Systems Therapy," written by Florence W. Kaslow, A. Rodney Nurse, and Peggy Thompson, warrants our attention. The authors describe three case studies through the lens of a variety of FST interventions that address "EMDR's Role in Breaking the Couples Impasse," "EMDR used to Facilitate Effective Co-parenting During a Divorce," and "EMDR Used in a Transgenerational Transmission Process." The authors provide an articulate discourse on the benefits of integrating EMDR with FST interventions in their case studies (see Kaslow et al., 2002). As Kaslow et al. explain,

> Because, understandably, therapy with couples tends to focus on the couple's history and the partners' stated views of their difficulties, individual background experiences undermining the couple's relationship are unlikely to be extensively explored, sometimes because of the need to cope with an immediate family crisis. EMDR provides an approach for quickly locating emotional blocks and trauma. In addition, it assists people with more fully experiencing pockets of affect and locating the often mistaken cognitive belief statement connected with the original experiences. They can then change the cognition to correspond with current situations that are similar in content or context to the original trauma.
>
> (p. 312)

Finally, in his 2007 Foreword in the *Handbook of EMDR and Family Therapy Processes*, Daniel Siegel further echoes my belief in the power of integrating EMDR and FST when he notes,

> EMDR and family systems therapy can be described as a powerful approach to facilitating integration within and among individuals. It is hypothesized

that the brains of individuals with traumatic histories may have impairments in the capacity to develop integrative patterns of firing. These patterns may be associated with unresolved issues and the disorganizing states of mind following painful loss and trauma. Using EMDR within a couples and family context catalyzes and integrates this neurobiological information and helps the client move towards states of security.

(p. xvi)

I encourage my readers to consult other essays in this publication such as "The Integration of EMDR and Family Systems Therapy," to see how Louise Maxfield, Florence W. Kaslow, and Francine Shapiro integrate specific FST models such as Structural Family Therapy, Experiential Therapy, Contextual Therapy, Bowenian Theory, and Integrative Family Therapy with EMDR; as well as Nancy J. Smyth's and A Desmond Poole's 2002 essay "EMDR and Cognitive-Behavioral Therapy: Exploring Convergence and Divergence." These authors thoughtfully advocate for the potency of integrating EMDR with FST, as noted by Siegel in his Preface.

I would also like to bring to the attention of my readers an insightful 2017 presentation, "EMDR with Couples and Families: Integrating EMDR Therapy with Relational Enhancement Therapy." In this presentation, Lisa Johnson and Margaret Moore explore the integration of EMDR with another FST modality, namely, Relationship Enhancement Therapy (RE). To my knowledge, the unique component of their approach in utilizing EMDR is that the individuals in the case studies are actually providing the bilateral stimulation (BLS) on one another with the therapist navigating the process. Johnson and Moore carefully guide their audience to an understanding of RE, an empathic modality intended to help couples actively hear the "other," resolve conflicts, and problem-solve in an effort to invoke both intrapersonal and interpersonal change. They also recognize the all-important neurobiological underpinnings of trauma EMDR, and they explore the neural basis for empathy as well as the neurobiological and clinical implications of BLS (discussed in Chapters 3 and 4 of this book). Johnson and Moore address their components of case selection and implementation (i.e., commitment to the relationship, the absence of violence, the presence of trust, and assessing the need for individual EMDR distinct from the need of EMDR in the couples system). They attend to the ethical responsibility of the EMDR therapist in preparing their clients for conjoint therapy, for example, screening for dissociation, reviewing orientation and informed consent, establishing safety, providing psychoeducation, and carefully following Francine Shapiro's eight-phase protocol (as discussed in Chapter 3). Johnson and Moore offer the videos of two case studies in which they take their audience through the integration of EMDR and RE which demonstrates some positive results for the couples. In the end, the presenters are responsible in recognizing the research needed to document the effectiveness of their model (Johnson and Moore, 2017).

In the present chapter, I will focus on a particularly integrated and client-centered FST model, the Metaframeworks perspective, which, as I mentioned earlier in this chapter, has seldom been researched or utilized from a clinical perspective *specifically* to enhance the effectiveness of EMDR in healing psychological trauma in family systems. Assuming that most of my readers have less familiarity with the Metaframeworks perspective, I will summarize its major concepts and assumptions, including the theories of the human condition; constraints; perspectivism; isomorphism; and the therapeutic alliance. Since I assume that my readers have already acquired a greater awareness of the EMDR protocol, I will address the theoretical and practical applications of the Metaframeworks perspective in an effort to establish an isomorphic presence with the theoretical and practical applications of EMDR. In addition, I will summarize the all-important multicultural, spiritual, and gender-specific conversations that the Metaframeworks perspective "brings to the table." During this journey, I will interweave segments of my sessions with a couple as an illustration of a family system in which both partners experience psychological trauma and other mental health diagnoses such as Attention Deficit Hyperactivity Disorder (ADHD), anxiety, and depression to concretize the parallel theoretical and practical threads of these modalities in assessing, treating, and evaluating the effects of constraints which are often informed by trauma.

Before I can begin my basic exposition of the Metaframeworks model, however, I need to acquaint the reader with some of the details of the case study that I will be utilizing. Given that this case study is not presented as *evidence* of the efficacy of my approach but, rather, as an *illustration* of how it works, I have taken the liberty of adding a small number of fictional details to fill in the gaps and render my account more coherent. However, I stayed within the parameters of the language used by the couple in order to avoid the trap of re-writing their narratives that they presented in session.

Evelyn and Andrew, an unmarried childless Caucasian couple in their early fifties, live in a residential home in Connecticut. They are both gainfully employed and both were previously married. They each presented with anxiety and minor depression in both their professional and personal lives that weighed heavily on their relationship. Evelyn reported that she felt overwhelmed by her work schedule and invisible when it came to connecting with Andrew's family of origin, friends, and independent social activities. In essence, Evelyn clearly felt that she was excluded from many aspects of Andrews' life and was simply not being "heard" by Andrew. Evelyn also reported that she felt that she was often acquiescing to Andrew's daily schedule which resulted in having little "quality time" to explore her individual interests as well as little "quality time" with her partner. Andrew reported that he was overwhelmed by his work schedule, that he was experiencing a lack of motivation and an inability to focus on one project at a time, and was clearly disturbed by what he coined his "lazy" side. Andrew also expressed frustration regarding Evelyn's lack of interest in participating in many of his favorite activities, her constant articulation of not being "heard," and not being in what Evelyn called a "real" partnership, as well as her complaints of not having enough "quality time" with him. Both Evelyn and Andrew also reported that they were experiencing escalating conflictual communication patterns as well as a lack of equanimity and emotional and physical intimacy in their partnership. Both reported, however, that they were committed to preserving their partnership and trying to find solutions to reconcile what they perceived as their respective frustrations, unmet needs, and differences.

Fundamental to our success as competent therapists practicing under the umbrella of postmodernism is an awareness and appreciation of the complexity of the human condition. As a Marriage and Family Therapist and AAMFT Approved Supervisor, I engage in a systems approach to identify, assess, and treat the complexities of the human condition. Thinking systemically, I strive to place the complexity of data into a relational context—identifying patterns, sequences, and redundancies that appear across the different systemic levels, referring back to my early training. I provided an individual consult with both Evelyn and Andrew in an effort to afford each of them an opportunity to share information that they might otherwise be uncomfortable doing in the couple session. Fortunately, there appeared to be no secrets within the couple subsystem that would compromise the couple or the therapeutic alliance. Given the complexities that presented in my couple within the human condition and the systems frame, my thinking about treatment in relational terms was naturally informed by the integrative approach of the Metaframeworks perspective that I first encountered during my years of training as a AAMFT supervisor.

My hypothesis regarding the couple subsystem was formed by many strategies. As a systemic thinker, I first assessed what their presenting problems were and when their problems started by asking the most obvious questions such as, "When did you notice the problems?" and "What was different in your lives when the problems started?" Secondly, I asked the couple whether there were times when the presenting problems were less apparent, and when they were more severe. Thirdly, I asked the couple if they had previous therapy in an attempt to solve their previous concerns, trying to ascertain what worked and what did not. I also thoroughly assessed the coping skills and resources that each possessed considering how that might contribute to any perceived imbalance in the relationship and how, as their therapist, I could encourage the development of these resources. I remembered the words of William M. Pinsof from his 1995 book *Integrated Problem-Centered Therapy: A Synthesis of Family, Individual and Biological Therapies*: "Identifying presenting problems and attempted solutions details the problem cycle. These first two steps are fundamentally behavioral: they are concerned with the sequential behaviors of the key system members in regard to the presenting problems" (p. 172).

The information that I gained from my initial inquiry with the couple guided me to administer an inclusive and "cost-effective" set of intake, screening, and diagnostic tools including the Beck's Anxiety and Depression Inventories; the Couples Satisfaction Scale Index (CSI-16); the Brief Accessibility Responsiveness and Engagement Scale (BARE); The Structural Clinical Interview, based on the Diagnostic and Statistical Manual of Mental Disorders (DSM-V); the Impact of Event Scale—Revised (IES-R); the PTSD Checklist Civilian Version (PCL-C); the Clinical Administered PTSD Scale for Adults (CAPS); the Traumatic History Questionnaire (THQ); and the Dissociative Experiences Scale (DES). The result of this inquiry was that Evelyn and Andrew's multiple, and frequently evolving relational presenting problems, were largely informed by their respective families of origin, their individual life experiences, and in particular, their psychological traumas, which they were initially reticent to face or discuss. It was here that I realized the necessity of establishing a safe and deep therapeutic alliance (see Chapter 3) with both the individuals and the couple. Some clinicians, theorists, and academics might argue that it is better to have one therapist treat the couple while engaging other therapists to treat each individual separately. However, this has proven less effective for me when working with couples suffering from psychological trauma. Pinsof, when describing the direct therapist system, in particular the middle phase, explains, "it is usually better for the same therapist to conduct the conjoint and individual sessions with members of the same patient system. This increases coordination of efforts, minimizes redundancy and fragmentation, and tends to keep all the 'therapies' focused on the presenting problems" (1995, p. 136).

I continued my integrated approach, as discussed in Chapter 4, by exploring the couples' attachment styles. After administering assessment tools for attachment issues and the genogram as noted below, both Evelyn's and Andrew's attachment styles proved to be insecure. While Evelyn demonstrated an insecure attachment style, specifically an ambivalent one, Andrew also demonstrated an insecure attachment style, dissimilar from Evelyn's in that it was an avoidant attachment style. While Evelyn, for example, never attached due to the inconsistent yet intrusive behavior of her mother, who worked many hours and sent her daughter to live with extended family members, Andrew attached to neither parent, instead forming attachments with his paternal grandparents, only to have them retire far away when Andrew was nine years of age. Creating awareness in the couple of their respective attachment styles seemed to elicit a better understanding and compassion for the "other's" ineffective communication styles, reactivity, and desired level of intimacy.

At this juncture, I administered the genogram (as discussed in Chapter 4). The genogram proved an effective tool in re-affirming their attachment issues and in identifying the repetition of dysfunctional systemic intergenerational patterns as well as identifying the psychological traumas suffered by Evelyn and Andrew. Evelyn, for example, had suffered from abandonment and from emotional abuse and neglect throughout most of her childhood after her parents divorced as she was constantly being moved into impoverished circumstances with members of her extended family. Evelyn reported that she "walked through her childhood feeling like Cinderella," always seeming invisible in her extended family. Her adult life proved equally unstable, married to an unpredictable and often emotionally abusive alcoholic spouse. As in many relationships where one partner uses alcohol or drugs, Evelyn demonstrated enabling and codependent tendencies. After the loss of his grandparents, Andrew became an alcoholic, and his Internal Family Systems (IFS) firefighter *part*, the part which puts out the pain followed Andrew until his first marriage when he started his recovery. However, Andrew carried the constant feeling of "not being good enough" and of being an underachiever, cognitions perpetuated by his parents, and by his spouse of many years who informed him that "she really never felt present in the marriage," and that she "never really loved him," a continuation of the psychological betrayal trauma that he was suffering from. Thankfully, Andrew continued his sobriety in spite of the loss of his wife and had maintained thirty years of sobriety when Andrew and Evelyn sought counseling.

After several collaborative discussions with the couple, Evelyn and Andrew developed an awareness that their difficulties in the present as a couple were informed by potent attachment issues and earlier psychological trauma as well as by negative beliefs about themselves and dysfunctional communications patterns, negative emotions, and sensations perpetuated by their respective childhood and adult experiences.

I continued the integrated process of enhancing the EMDR protocol with the couple by providing psychoeducation on IFS and working through their Internal Family Systems. It became obvious that neither Evelyn nor Andrew were leading with a differentiated-Self. Both Evelyn and Andrew demonstrated extreme exiles/burdened parts as well as extreme protective parts, i.e., managers and firefighters. After working with each individually and at times conjointly to lower the extremity of their internal parts (e.g., having these extreme *parts* converse with the *parts* of the differentiated-Self that they had such as compassion, curiosity, creativity, and courage), Evelyn and Andrew began to acquire a better understanding or wisdom of their parts or aspects of their personalities. It was at this point that both Evelyn and Andrew started to recognize the other components or "C's" of "Self" leadership that they were lacking such as clarity (or wisdom) calmness, confidence, and connectedness. Bringing this awareness and development back into couple therapy proved fruitful in sympathizing with the "other" and understanding how the interaction of their internal parts in specific sequences and styles mimicked the styles and patterns that characterized their relationship as a couple, a thorough investigation of which is beyond the purview of this book.

At this stage of integration, I began the process of enhancing safety within Evelyn and Andrew through the practice of mindfulness (as discussed in Chapters 3 and 4) before beginning the EMDR protocol to address their psychological trauma. In a collaborative journey which took place during their individual and couple sessions, I first provided psychoeducation on the importance of building a tool-kit of self-soothing techniques, engaging in the practice of mindfulness, and the installation of a safe/calm place, part of the Preparation phase of the EMDR protocol, as discussed in Chapter 3. During our sessions, we engaged in the practice of many mindfulness exercises, some of which are presented in this book, and the couple was encouraged to practice these exercises consistently between their individual and couple sessions. Evelyn and

Andrews's choice of a safe/calm place was successfully installed and proved to be mostly successful as I continued to assess throughout the EMDR process.

While I utilized the EMDR Case Conceptualization assessment, developed by Dr. Helene Stoller, my EMDRIA approved consultant in training (see Appendix 5) and initiated the integrated EMDR neurobiological protocol separately with Evelyn and Andrew, I continued to work with the couple on a bi-monthly basis to assess and track their presenting problems. By this point, Evelyn and Andrew were engaged as active participants in sharing the results of their individual therapeutic treatments with EMDR. This relational component proved to be a powerful tool in helping both Evelyn and Andrew understand the "other's" reactivity and inability to self-regulate due to their respective psychological traumas. At this juncture, the couples' ability to listen with curiosity to their respective internal *parts* improved and lowered their reactivity towards one another and enhanced their mutual compassion.

The Metaframeworks Perspective

We are now in a position to investigate the Metaframeworks perspective in earnest. The Greek prefix *meta-* means, literally, "after." After I have looked at each of six trees separately, I can step back and consider them as a unit. When I look at how they compete with one another for sunshine and how they collectively use the soil, for example, I am exercising a meta-perspective on the six trees.

The inventors of the Metaframeworks perspective, whom we shall meet later in this section, thought about the myriad of useful therapeutic strategies available to the practitioner and judiciously culled crucial elements that those strategies have in common. They then constructed six "meta-frameworks," namely, organization, sequences, mind, development, gender, and culture. As we shall see, they then brought to bear within those metaframeworks a suite of analytic concepts and a careful delineation of basic levels, and the Metaframeworks perspective was born.

This approach is best described as a common factors approach based on a biopsychosocial continuum, i.e., biology, person, relationship, family, community, and society that considers multi-leveled human systems for assessment and treatment, i.e., organization, sequences, mind, development, gender, and culture, which is precisely what the authors mean by the term *metaframeworks*, or domains that serve as a lens through which a family problem can be examined and resolved.

From my perspective, the Metaframeworks approach honors the complexity of human systems in ways that purist, single-perspective models simply cannot, namely by providing the tools for therapists to quickly and effectively organize the highly complex data presented by couples and families in order to develop a comprehensive treatment plan. As such, the Metaframeworks perspective enhances the efficacy of EMDR when working with couples like Evelyn and Andrew suffering from the comorbidity of psychological trauma and other

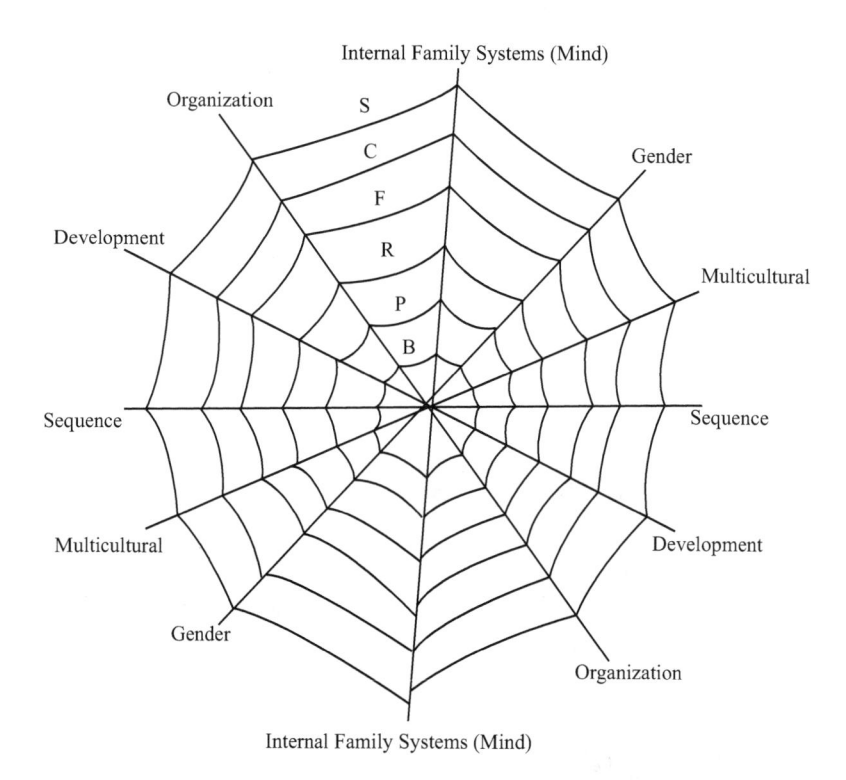

The letters in the figure stand for the levels of biopsychosocial continuum:
B = biology, P = person, R = relationship, F = family, C = community, and S = society.

Figure 5.1 The Web of Constraints

(Reproduced from Breunlin et al., 1992) [Reprinted with permission from John Wiley & Sons]

mental health diagnoses, and which manifested as numerous presenting problems (Figure 5.1).

There are several assumptions within the Metaframeworks perspective that inform my thinking about assessment and treatment in relational terms. One of the major assumptions is the "theory of constraints." Rooted in one of the leading principles from cybernetics known as negative explanation (Bateson, 1972), the theory of constraints espouses that clients could solve their problems if they were not unduly constrained from doing so. I find this assumption particularly helpful when treating trauma in internal and external family systems since this assumption reflects a non-deficit and a non-resistant-based view of human nature, implying that with some guidance, clients and therapists have the potential to tap into their resources and strengths to help remove constraints (Breunlin, 1999). Other critical presuppositions of the

Metaframeworks perspective that inform my thinking and trauma practice in relational terms explore the concepts of power and "perspectivism." According to Breunlin et al. (1997),

> Perspectivism purports that 'reality does really exist out there,' but we cannot know it objectively because our perceptual apparatus and our system of internal parts provide incomplete access to it and distort any data we receive from it. Perspectivism also holds that while we cannot completely really know reality, we can work to achieve better approximations to of it.
>
> (p. 33)

"I believe," continues Breunlin, "that the theory of constraints, albeit incomplete, does offer a better application of reality than any *one* of the models of therapy" (p. 33, italics mine). As a trauma clinician, I take great solace that we can work towards a better approximation of reality, a view of the mind based on multiplicity where the Self is the internal leader and mediator for various parts (Breunlin, 1999; Schwartz, 1997; see discussion in Chapter 4).

Conducting therapy using the multi-leveled and multidimensional perspective of the Metaframeworks approach provides me with a conceptual and recursive schema to efficiently organize and manage the complexity of the human condition, as will be seen clinically below in working through a multileveled biopsychosocial system and six metaframeworks/domains to remove constraints in a couple subsystem. I will also demonstrate how an FST model, such as the Metaframeworks perspective, enhances the neurobiological EMDR protocol since, like many of the concepts discussed, parallel concepts that exist in the EMDR protocol such as Shapiro's Adaptive Information Processing (AIP), which posits that much of psychopathology is due to maladaptive coding of traumatic experiences (which, in the language of the Metaframeworks perspective, can easily be translated into constraints), and the incomplete processing of traumatic events (as discussed in Chapter 3).

The Six Constraints in the Biopsychosocial System and the Six Constraints Within the Metaframeworks

At this juncture, it is important for my readers to recall the six constraints in the biopsychosocial system and the six constraints within the metaframeworks/domain already introduced, whose general meaning as well as the meaning for my couple will be codified in this section.

Individuals are nested within larger units that are, in turn, located within yet larger contexts. We must recognize the evermore encompassing progression from the individual, to the nuclear family, and on to the extended family, the family's social context, the historical and cultural context, the current national social systems, and finally the international system (Breunlin et al., 1992).

As Breunlin et al. note,

> Isomorphism allows us to use the same concepts to describe different levels of systems. Therefore, we can expect to find pattern, organization, and development at each level of a system. Metaframeworks are our vehicle for the specific ideas that therapists need in working with human systems. Each metaframework classifies a domain of ideas and organizes it into metapatterns. The domains derive from the considerations of systems theory. *Sequences* and *organization* are fundamental properties of systems, just as *development* is fundamental to living systems. To understand a human system, we must also have the knowledge about its objects—the people who make up the system—and we gain this knowledge through the domain of *internal process*. We have found it impossible to understand human systems without serious consideration of *gender*, the core attribute that distinguishes males from females. Finally, at the broadest level, human systems are defined by *culture*.
>
> (pp. 44–45)

The Six Constraints in the Biopsychosocial System

In his 1999 article "Toward a Theory of Constraints," Breunlin codifies the systemic intent of the Metaframeworks perspective as discussed and addresses the concepts of constraints when he explains,

> Grounded in the cybernetic concept of negative explanation, the theory of constraints examines how human systems are kept from solving problems. To identify constraints, the therapist must know where to look for them and what to look for. The theory proposes that constraints exist among the levels of a biopsychosocial system, which include [1] biology, [2] person, [3] relationship, [4] family, [5] community and [6] society.
>
> (p. 365)

Constraints in biology (1) are often missed since therapists rarely explore them, with the exception of the obvious ones that often present in my clinical practice (e.g., obesity, heart problems, kidney issues, chronic pain, migraine headaches, chronic digestive conditions such as irritable bowel syndrome [IBS] and reflux). Missing biological constraints can impede the therapeutic process. In his 1995 book *Integrative Problem-Centered Therapy: A Synthesis of Family, Individual, and Biological Therapies*, Pinsof explains, "Biological processes are most likely to play an implicit role in the following presenting problems: substance abuse, major mental illnesses [i.e., psychological trauma], and failures in normal functioning with a clear organic base" (pp. 172–173). To avoid missing the more subtle constraints in this system, I always offer van der Kolk's theory that "the body keeps the score," and explain to my clients how they can become "flooded" with a tsunami of more potent somatic complaints after experiencing a trauma. It was at this juncture that I began to witness constraints among the levels of the biopsychosocial system in the couple starting with the level of biology. While Evelyn, for example, suffered from constant fatigue, and chronic joint and back pain, Andrew suffered from back pain as well as a chronic digestive condition, acid reflux disorder, many of which may have resulted from their psychological traumas and the chronic anxiety and depression that followed. They came to realize how these biological constraints were negatively impacting their desire and ability to communicate in "loving" ways.

As Breunlin notes in his 1999 article, "Constraints at the level of person [2] are traditionally associated with the psychology of the self, particularly how one experiences self; how self makes, interprets, and experiences meaning and emotion; and how the self-constructs a blueprint for action" (p. 370). When addressing the level of the person (2), I find utilizing the Internal Family Systems (IFS) model to be the most telling in the identification of constraints. In fact, one might argue that much of the language used throughout the Metaframeworks perspective reflects that of the IFS model, introduced in Chapter 4, a model which also enhances the effectiveness of the EMDR protocol. During my sessions with the couple, it was apparent that constraints on this level existed for both partners. Evelyn's experience of Self, for example, was compromised. She admitted being abandoned and dismissed as a child as well as during her first marriage to an alcoholic spouse, neither getting her emotional needs satisfied nor feeling safe in any relationship. In the couple subsystem, Evelyn's sense of self was further compromised. Evelyn felt insecure since she earned less money than Andrew, was not included in many aspects of his life, was informed by Andrew that they would never marry, and always felt that her lack of attention to her appearance (i.e., wearing makeup and dressing in a more feminine manner) was a constant source of disappointment for Andrew. Andrew's sense of self was also compromised by his distress at having been abandoned by both of his parents and grandparents, his guilt from resorting to alcohol as a coping mechanism, having a diagnosis of ADHD, considering himself an underachiever, and from the betrayal trauma inflicted upon him by his first spouse. In addition, Andrew felt compromised by the criticism he received from Evelyn that he could never stay on task, had too many interests outside of the home, and demonstrated little emotional availability.

It became clear that both Evelyn and Andrew were experiencing anxiety, mild depression, anger, sadness, and grief, constraints at the level of person. As Pinsof so aptly recognizes, "In understanding the emotion system underlying the problem cycle, the critical issues are identifying which emotions are present and which emotions are missing and the extent to which what is present or what is missing facilitates or hinders problem-solving" (p. 176). In the case of Evelyn and Andrew, their frequent and intense emotions were hindering their capacity to communicate and connect.

When investigating the level of Relationship (3), I focus on the couple, exploring their rules, roles, hierarchies, patterns of communication, emotions, intimacy, and equity as well as the politics of gender and culture. Evelyn and Andrew experienced many constraints on this level. Evelyn felt that the rules were mostly determined by Andrew, but perhaps not always intentionally. She did, however, feel stuck in a "one-down" position since Andrew made more money, and they both equated money with power. As systems thinkers I am sure we are all aware that money often factors into the negative power dynamics of many couples that come to us for therapy. Evelyn's "one-down" position was further bolstered by her being placed in charge of all of the domestic tasks on top of her challenges at work. Evelyn's resulting emotion was one of feeling overwhelmed. All of these constraints further complicated the couples' ability to communicate, to address each other's emotional needs, and to achieve equity, thus removing the chance of experiencing emotional and physical intimacy.

The Family level (4) is a core level where, in my view, differentiation, enmeshment, fusion, and cutoff are the main constraints, as discussed in Chapter 4. In this biopsychosocial level, the couple experienced opposite constraints. Since Evelyn had experienced an ambivalent attachment style in her family of origin, the natural progression manifested as insecurity and reactivity within the couple subsystem. Andrew, by contrast, demonstrated an avoidant attachment style that morphed into intermittent, but intense, bouts of fear, frustration, and mild depression. As a result, emotions such as fear, love, rejection, and irritability continued to appear during the initial and intermediary stages of both individual and couple therapy.

Regarding the location of constraints found in the level of Community (5), my goal is to access the family's safety, educational, medical, and financial needs and to explore with them their access to community resources. I am sure my readers have all experienced how these needs can be blocked by lack of access to a robust social services system. The couple, Evelyn and Andrew, lacked constraints in this biopsychosocial level since as a couple, while not considered to be "well off," both were securely employed, had access to good medical insurance, experienced safety in the couple subsystem in the traditional "physical" sense. As such, the couple lacked the need for traditional community services.

As evident in the many prejudices, norms, and values that exist in our Society (6) around divorce, religion, politics, gender identification, and ethnicity, this level poses a host of problems in unraveling constraints. Although the couple was on the same page regarding religion, politics, and ethnicity, the constraints around divorce and marriage weighed heavily in their partnership since Evelyn believed in the importance of marriage in the eyes of society and felt less important in her status as a partner rather than as a spouse. Andrew, on the other hand, experienced a sense of pain and betrayal in his previous marriage and had no interest in marrying again.

The Six Constraints Within the Metaframeworks

Just as there are six constraints in the biopsychosocial system, there are also six constraints within the metaframework or domain. For the sake of clarity in what follows, so that my readers do not confuse the six constraints in the biopsychosocial system with those in the metaframeworks or domains, the former have been (and will continue to be) consistently designated with Arabic numerals (1)–(6) while the latter are introduced with lower-case letters (a)–(f). In their 1992 book *Metaframeworks: Transcending the Models of Family Therapy*, Breunlin et al., clarify the rationale of working with the six domains:

> First, we use systems theory to describe human systems as complex, multilevel entities. Second, we set forth presuppositions concerning the human condition, and we hold them constant throughout our work. Third, to understand the specifics of the human condition as it is related to therapy, we use six domains. Each one contains ideas pertinent to the human condition, at the level of theory and/or knowledge about it. In the domain of development, for example, we would expect to find ideas about biological, individual, relational and family development.
>
> (p. 23)

As Breunlin et al. continue,

> Metaframeworks are our vehicle for the specific ideas that therapists need in working with human systems. Each metaframework classifies a domain of ideas and organizes into metapatterns. The domains derive from the consideration of systems theory. Sequences and organization are fundamental properties of systems, just as development is fundamental to living systems. To understand a human system, we must also have knowledge about its objects—the people who make up the systems—and we gain the knowledge through the domain of internal process. We have found it impossible to understand human systems without serious consideration of gender, the core attribute that distinguishes males from females. Finally, at the broadest level, human systems are defined by culture. Other domains could have been included in our perspective, but we have limited our scheme to these six domains because they map our clinical experience so well.
>
> (pp. 44–45)

The six frameworks/domains of (a) organization, (b) sequences, (c) mind, (d) development, (e) gender, and (f) culture assist in constraint identification. Breunlin further explains that "combining the levels of metaframeworks creates a web of constraints, the complexity of which determines how difficult it will be to solve a given problem. The theory of constraint offers an *integrative* and pragmatic approach to therapy while simultaneously honoring the complexity of human systems" (p. 365, italics mine).

As an underlying map, then, the Metaframeworks perspective approach recognizes that constraints exist among the levels of this biopsychosocial system, i.e., (1) biology, (2) person, (3) relationship, (4) family, (5) community, and

(6) society, as identified by Breunlin. Once we know where to look for constraints, the other piece centers around being aware of what to look for and how to label and identify the constraints at any applicable level. The six frameworks/domains assist the therapist as to where to find the constraints (i.e., (a) organization, (b) sequences, (c) mind, (d) development, (e) gender, and (f) culture) and imply, based upon assumptions such as isomorphism (discussed earlier in the chapter), that the constraints can be removed with the help of a competent therapist (Breunlin et al.).

In his 1997 article "Toward a Theory of Constraints," Breunlin speaks to (a) the organization metaframework: "The organization metaframework examines two core constructs: boundaries and leadership. When system boundaries and their leadership function effectively, each system level will show balance and harmony and the system will function well" (p. 372). As previously discussed, regarding the biopsychosocial level of Relationship (3), Evelyn and Andrew suffered from constraints in the area of roles and rules which is always an accurate predicator of poor boundaries in Family System Therapist. Furthermore, regarding the construct of leadership, as already discussed, both Andrew and Evelyn bought into the construct given their correlation of money with power. As Pinsof further specifies, "Organization encompasses balance, harmony and leadership (p. 10). As Pinsof continues, "To have balance and harmony, a system must have leadership" (p. 10). According to Pinsof, "*Balance* refers to influence, access to resources, and level of responsibility. *Harmony* deals with the extent to which the system members 'cooperate,' are willing to sacrifice some of their individual interests for the greater good, care about one another and feel valued by the larger system, and have clear boundaries that allow a balance between belonging and separateness (Breunlin et al., 1992, p. 10). In the end, as Pinsof notes, "Poor leadership constrains balance and harmony, and imbalance and disharmony constrain effective leadership" (p. 10). And this was clearly the case within the couple subsystem, since Evelyn and Andrew presented with many constraints in the metaframework of organization, i.e., Evelyn and Andrew's lack of access to resources, lack of willingness to sacrifice individual interests, a lack of a balance of belonging and separateness, and a discrepancy in what each of them perceived as an appropriate level of responsibility in the couple, as discussed earlier in this chapter.

Regarding (b), according to Breunlin (1999), "The sequences metaframework uses four classes of sequences: brief face-to-face sequences, sequences of daily routine [that go from a day to a week], sequences that ebb and flow over a period of time from a week to a year, and transgenerational sequences [that go from one generation to the next]" (p. 372). Evelyn experienced several constraints in these four areas of communication, having "never been heard," never having her emotional needs met by her parents, being dismissed in her previous marriage by an alcoholic spouse and by Andrew whom she perceived as just too busy and unfocused to hear what she was saying. Andrew presented with similar constraints in these four areas of communication which began during his childhood with absent parents and later absent grandparents and continued in his ineffective dialogues with Evelyn throughout their partnership.

As for (c), according to Breunlin (1999), "The metaframework of the mind captures the domain of ideas about mental process in human systems. Manifestations of this mental process exist at all levels of the biopsychosocial system. The biochemistry of the brain can constrain mental process, as can meaning-making schemas of the person" (p. 373). As Breunlin continues, "Of particular value is the principle of multiplicity, which asserts that all levels of the mind are composed of parts that can become polarized and extreme and, therefore, generate constraints of the mind" (p. 373). The domain of the mind does not accept a "monolithic" view of the mind, but instead, see it as a series of "*parts*" (Breunlin et al., 1992). This domain, when working with individuals, embraces the language of the Internal Family Systems (IFS), as discussed in Chapter 4. The benefit of the IFS modality, when working with couples, is that it provides the therapist with the ability to see how each of the client's internal parts may be affecting the problem in the external family system. I focused the next session on psycho-educating the couple on the meaning of IFS in individual and couples therapy. In her 2013 essay "Self in Relationship: An Introduction to IFS Couple Therapy," Herbine-Blank notes, "Internal family systems therapy (IFS) invites people first to learn how to be in a loving relationship with themselves and, from that state, to attempt a heartfelt connection with their intimate partner" (Herbine-Blank, p. 55). She goes on to explain,

> We work with the internal system much as we would work with an external system, learning about the roles and protective functions of parts, supporting the development of relationships between parts, and between parts and Self, and then helping our clients to access vulnerable young parts who carry the burdens of relational trauma. As the internal system shifts we can usually observe positive effects on external relationships as well. In brief we see the external mirroring the internal. We always keep in mind that the painful polarizations, fears, conflict, rage and withdrawal that we see between partners are also occurring internally between the parts of each client. The art of couple work in IFS lies in balancing in-depth individual IFS work with a focus on the relationship. This entails a variety of strategies: asking one person to go inside while supporting the other one to remain engaged and present; then moving back to external relational work and teaching the couple to speak for parts, listen from Self and try on new ways of behaving that foster differentiation, individuality and connection.
> (Herbine-Blank, p. 58)

As Evelyn's extreme exiled parts (fear, abandonment, shame), acquired from her childhood and adult traumatic experiences, were heard by Andrew, who began to connect with his own exiled parts (fear abandonment, shame, and what he termed an inherent "lazy streak"), which were heard in turn by Evelyn, the couple began to experience compassion and were able to stay present. As a result, Evelyn gradually began to self-regulate her angry and critical parts towards Andrew and communicate more effectively. In turn, when Andrew's extreme protective parts (i.e., fear of abandonment / "keeping her at bay" and shame of being an underachiever) were witnessed by Evelyn, she demonstrated compassion for Andrew's distressed parts. As a result, Andrew began to see Evelyn as compassionate and caring, and he responded by embracing more equity and intimacy in the partnership. Thus, by working through Evelyn's and Andrew's individual parts and having them serve as the other's witness, the couples' communication improved. Instead of speaking and listening from their extreme parts, the couple began to speak and listen from their more differentiated Selves, attuned and empathetic.

When it comes to (d), Breunlin (1999) explains, "The developmental metaframework examines the competencies required for each level of a system, and the system as a whole, to function effectively and to develop appropriately. Constraints emerge when any level of the system is not functioning in a developmentally appropriate way" (p. 372). "When development expectations are not clear," continues Breunlin, "one or more family members may show a developmental oscillation in which that person acts older and/or younger than is age appropriate" (p. 372).

A developmental oscillation proved to be a constraint since both Evelyn and Andrew were forced to act older and younger than age-appropriate within their communication styles. Andrew, through no fault of his own, was simultaneously placed in the younger role given his problems with focusing and his perception of having a "lazy streak" (i.e., being an underachiever) as well as being placed in the older role of being the higher wage earner, while Evelyn was simultaneously placed in the older role as both an enabler and "parental figure," not dissimilar to the role she was placed during her first marriage with an alcoholic spouse. At the same time, she was placed in the younger role of insecurity, being in the position of the lower wage earner and not having her emotional needs met. Both Andrew and Evelyn were caught in an emotional whipsaw; they were each split into two age-inappropriate roles and forced back-and-forth between them.

On (e), the gender metaframework, note Breunlin's assertion that

> The different ways that males and females are socialized and their differential access to and exercise of power can create constraints at all levels. Gender is a biological reality and a major construct of personhood. The politics of gender deeply affect relationships, and gender-prescribed roles can severely impact how a family functions. In communities and at the societal level, the social construction of gender has a deep impact on men and women. Work with couples and families must take into account the respective level of gender awareness of all family members, and therapy often increases a couple's mutual awareness of and ability to have gender-balanced relationship.
>
> (1999, p. 372)

Feminist critique informs my work as a systems trauma therapist. I often find myself functioning in the role of an educator exploring the different ways that men and women have been socialized, especially regarding patriarchal organization, where, according to Breunlin et al. (1992) "men unquestionably have more influence than women do in all sociopolitical areas" (p. 245). Clearly there was a constraint in this domain for Evelyn, who never attained access to education beyond high school or age-appropriate independence as a child and adolescent, witnessing both a dominant father figure and dominant males in her extended family. She was socialized to perform "woman's work" (cleaning and picking up after others during both her childhood and adulthood) and was forced by her family of origin and extended family to remain silent. This pattern would repeat itself during her first marriage with a substance-abusing spouse. And, as so often in our early couple sessions, Evelyn would remark about Andrew, "It's his work, his extracurricular activities, and plans that always come first. The domestic work always seems to fall on me even though we work the same hours."

Given that this gender reality is still with us in the twenty-first century, I often explore with my trauma survivors how they have attained access to power and how these processes are creating the small "t" or large "T" in their lives. These inequities can create constraints on all levels (e.g., biological, personhood, society, and community). Therefore I always make it a point to assess the level of gender awareness among my clients, encouraging all to take responsibility for accountability and change. I believe that it is essential for us to take a position against gender oppression and to establish relationships with an eye on gender equality based on equal amounts of influence and equal access to resources. As such, I have found it helpful to engage clients in a dialogue whereby each participant moves through stages of gender awareness, e.g., traditional patriarchal meaning (discussions of the cultural revolution), polarization (encouraging negotiation of balanced gender roles), transition (supporting and validating beliefs and clarifying new roles), and balance (supporting egalitarian potential for intimacy), wherein equity is reached (see Breunlin et al., 1992). Given that gender politics are so consumed by emotions related to long periods of neglect, especially in those suffering from trauma, I create a safe, stable, and transparent environment open for discussion, devoid of blame, shame, or any other kind of exploitation. This resonates, not only in the preparation phase of EMDR, but throughout the entire integration of EMDR and Metaframeworks, since when mutual respect, increased accountability, and open, transparent dialogue are present, constraints are more easily removed. This turned out to be the case with Evelyn and Andrew. Having developed a set of questions for Evelyn and Andrew, for example, which explored their own experiences, along with providing psychoeducation on patriarchal thinking (e.g., issues of gender [as discussed] which escalated for the couple during the 2016 U.S. presidential election). This dialogue allowed each partner to put themselves in the other's place, balancing the couple's extreme parts and explaining the benefits of increased equity and intimacy. As a result, Evelyn and Andrew achieved greater harmony and balance as a couple. I also used the following words delivered by the character of Atticus Finch from Harper Lee's novel *To Kill a Mockingbird* (also used in the classic 1960 movie of the novel and quoted by former President Barack Obama during his 2016 farewell speech) to close the deal: "you never really understand a person until you consider things from his [her] point of view, until you climb into his [her] skin and walk around in it."

Regarding (f), in the domain of culture, according to Breunlin,

> We draw our identity from simultaneous membership in a multitude of contexts that includes our ethnic and racial origins, our religious, regional, economic and educational, sexual preference and age contexts. In a mobile and transitioning society, our degree of involvement and acceptance in these contexts varies across levels through the processes of immigration and acculturation. These contexts can provide a sense of fit or lack of fit, the latter creating the potential for constraints.
>
> (1999, p. 372)

In their 2003 study "Complex Trauma in Children and Adolescents," the National Child Traumatic Stress Network (NCTSN), Alexandra Cook, Margaret Blaustein, Joseph Spinazzola, and Bessel van der Kolk (eds.) explain, "Different cultures have different concepts of family, in terms of who is a member, the roles and responsibilities of each member, and how involved family members are with different children" (p. 19). The authors of this study go on to note, "The chosen trauma treatment may be individualized to the family's needs, but yet may not fit with the family's cultural understanding of the child's role in the family system" (p. 19). If there are dissimilar stages of acculturation in the same family, a dichotomy around ethnic sensibility can occur leading to a further disconnect regarding their perceived cultural and ethnic identity (see www.NCTSNet.org).

Constraints for Evelyn and Andrew located in this domain were nonexistent regarding differences in cultural and ethnic identity. They both grew up in families whose cultural ties were to Western Europe. They were both a product of divorce and were both forced to live with extended family members. They presented with constraints, however, in the economic and educational realms. As mentioned, Evelyn's moderate poverty growing up as a child with little access to education placed her in a situation where she was unable to earn as much as Andrew, thus perceiving herself in a "one down" position. Andrew's lack of self-esteem due to what he coined his perception of being "a shameful underachiever" and former substance abuser created a potent constraint for him in this domain as well. Creating an awareness of these differences by having the couple communicate their narratives, therapeutic validating and normalizing of their feelings and working with their extreme burdened parts, proved effective in increasing the awareness of the "other," thus diminishing these constraints in the couple subsystem.

These six unique, flexible, and co-evolving metaframeworks/domains provide an invaluable lens in the hypothesis of systemic constraints. As a therapeutic system, the Metaframeworks perspective supports engaging in a collaborative process which is fluid in nature and constantly changing by way of constructing new meanings as to who we are, and with whom we are in conversation at any given moment. The collaborative stance, which co-evolves over time, the presence of a non-deficit view, the emphasis placed on caring, empathy, and validation, and an ability to meet our clients where they are, parallels the intent of the EMDR protocol. Furthermore, Metaframeworks' emphasis on obtaining a detailed client history, and discovering how patterns of relating and behaving can inform clients' actions and behaviors in the present and future, confirms an isomorphic relationship with Shapiro's eight phases of treatment, discussed in Chapter 4. Most importantly, when working with a couple where both partners experienced trauma, it became clearer to me from my experience working with the Metaframeworks perspective that trauma affects individuals and their partners in multifaceted ways. As we have seen, many constraints were located in the levels of the biopsychosocial system of Evelyn and Andrew as well as in the six metaframeworks. As a result, the couple relationship was impaired. Once Andrew and Evelyn became aware of these constraints, I was able to implement the blueprint for therapy, discussed in the next section. Individual, relational, and contextual variables needed to be addressed, and the Metaframeworks perspective proved to handle the complexities surrounding the effects of trauma given its multi-leveled and multidimensional frame and helped access the complexity of trauma and resulting constraints in the couples frame.

A Blueprint for Therapy

Another building block for the Metaframeworks perspective is a blueprint for therapy (Figure 5.2).

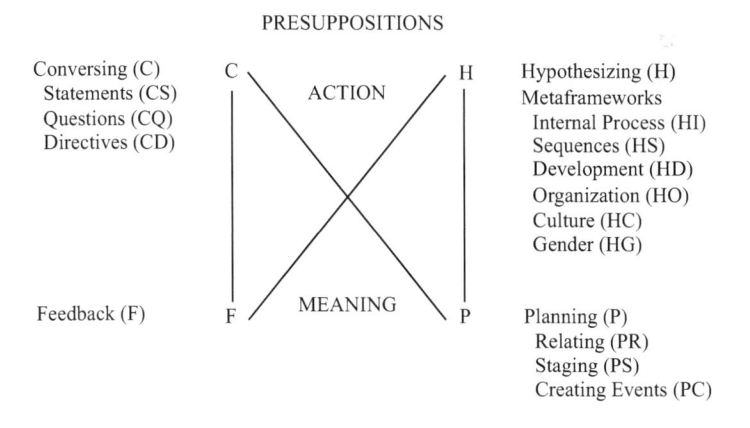

PRESUPPOSITIONS

Conversing (C)
Statements (CS)
Questions (CQ)
Directives (CD)

ACTION

Hypothesizing (H)
Metaframeworks
Internal Process (HI)
Sequences (HS)
Development (HD)
Organization (HO)
Culture (HC)
Gender (HG)

Feedback (F)

MEANING

Planning (P)
Relating (PR)
Staging (PS)
Creating Events (PC)

EXPERIENCE, DESCRIPTION, EXPLANATION

Figure 5.2 A Blueprint for Therapy
(Reproduced from Breunlin et al., 1992) [Reprinted with permission from John Wiley & Sons]

According to Breunlin, Schwartz, and Mac Kune-Karrer,

> The blueprint is nothing more than a set of guidelines for operationalizing the metaframeworks perspective in the actual conduct of therapy. Our presuppositions lead to a holistic view of human systems as multileveled entities, wherein each level influences and is influenced by the others and problems arise from the constraints imposed at one or more levels. We see change occurring through a collaborative effort between the therapist and the family to remove constraints.
>
> (1992, p. 281)

As the authors continue, "We identify four interrelated components that constitute the process of therapy: hypothesizing, planning, conversing and reading feedback. The four components are recursively related, so that therapists are constantly checking one against the others" (p. 287).

As the authors explain further,

> We define *hypothesizing*, as selecting a set of ideas drawn from one or more metaframeworks, which organizes and makes understandable specific feedback offered by the system. *Planning* is selecting a course of action for conducting therapy at any point. *Conversing* is deciding what to say to the family on a moment-to-moment basis. *Reading feedback* is observing and attributing meaning to the family's utterances and interactions in the context of therapy.
>
> (p. 287)

Expanding on these definitions, the authors consider *hypothesizing* as the conceptual and directional piece of therapy and a "conceptual exercise between therapist and family," such as conducting an interview and maintaining constant access to six conceptual domains depending on the client's feedback. For example, although we may open one domain, according to the client's feedback, we may have to navigate between domains if the family requires another domain to be opened. As such, hypothesizing, which depends on feedback, requires collaboration between the internal and external family systems (Breunlin et al., 1992).

Planning/Relating refers to the importance of the therapeutic relationship. *Planning/staging* refers to attending to how the therapeutic conversations are going and the flexibility to shift, and *Planning/creating events* centers around the therapists and collaborating as well as struggling with the family to remove constraints that limit their healthy functioning. Planning, in general, encompasses making choices in terms of which level of the biopsychosocial continuum to consider (i.e., biological, individual, subsystem, family, and larger systems levels) during any time when engaged in the *blueprint for therapy* (Breunlin et al.).

Conversing is another collaborative process in the *blueprint for therapy*. It is transparent, mutually connected, and a combination of "questions, statements, and directives" complementary with a therapist's style of relating that should be manifested in a genuine and caring way.

In their 1992 book, Breunlin et al. further expand on the nature of questions, statements, and directions by explaining:

> In the context of treatment we define a question as any sentence intended to elicit a response that will generate new or existing information. A Statement is a declarative sentence in which the therapist offers new or existing information to the system. A directive is an imperative sentence in which the therapist directs the system to do something.
>
> (p. 304)

Reading Feedback, another interrelated component in the blueprint for therapy, takes place throughout the therapeutic process. As Breunlin et al. note, "The utterances and interactions of a family takes place in the context of therapy and they constitute a form of feedback that must be read by the therapist and used to guide the progress of the therapy" (p. 307). As a guide for the therapeutic process, the therapist must also stay attuned to all the components at the same time, and refrain from incorporating feedback into hypothesizing and planning until the therapist and family are on the same page (Breunlin et al., 1992). In my experience, these four components share many aspects with Shapiro's Adaptive Information Processing (AIP) eight-phase modality in the EMDR neurological protocol, three-pronged strategy, and the role of the therapist (see Chapters 3 and 6).

Utilizing Breunlin and his colleagues' blueprint for therapy with Evelyn and Andrew proved productive. As Evelyn and Andrew were healing from their traumatic experiences by way of the EMDR protocol, which lowered their level of reactivity to one another and improved Andrews's ability to focus and remain on one task at a time, the couple's constraints in the biopsychosocial and metaframework/domain were also being addressed and processed in an integrated and collaborative way through constant hypothesis and navigation between their internal and external family systems. Having successfully joined with me after the first four sessions, as both individuals and as a couple, their sense of safety and trust in my therapeutic skills and in our collaborative journey proved meaningful. I made every attempt to professionally guide and protect Evelyn and Andrew every step of the way from their initial intake, I prioritized my therapeutic decision-making process based on evidence-based research, clinical skills, and teaching experience. At the same time, by remaining transparent and flexible throughout their treatment and especially during the Metaframeworks *blueprint*, going where they needed to go, and making certain that all constraints were addressed, the therapeutic process remained challenging yet manageable.

As mentioned in Chapters 3 and 4, I have always found *tracking* to be most helpful in managing any serious endeavor, but particularly when engaged in therapy that is complex, multileveled, multidimensional, integrated, and collaborative, that is, the very sort of integration of EMDR with other systemic modalities that this book champions. As we have seen, tracking is a vital and necessary component throughout both the Metaframeworks perspective and EMDR's eight-phase protocol. Moreover, it is the essence of any ethical and responsible approach to treating psychological trauma. My tracking work, for example, commenced during the intake process, continued through the stages of exploring attachment styles, conducting assessments, practicing mindfulness, working through the IFS model during every phase of the EMDR protocol and during the utilization of the Metaframeworks perspective, to enhance the effectiveness of EMDR for my clients. Clearly, in his 2010 book *The Mindful Therapist*, Daniel Siegel also recognizes the critical importance of the *integration* of tracking when he notes, "A crucial way that we stay present with our patients is to track what they are experiencing, moment by moment. This tracking involves communicating what they are experiencing in the here and now and being open with them so they can 'stay with' whatever arises in their awareness" (p. 136).

Mindfulness Redux

Continuing our discussion of his invaluable exploration of mindfulness from my previous chapter, we now turn to how Siegel takes us on a *mindful* journey, where we experience a "flow of energy" that guides us from the individual practice of contemporary mindfulness to what it means to be systemically mindful, a transformation from the "me" to "we." The focus of this odyssey is grounded in Siegel's mindful concepts of Presence, Attunement, and Resonance, thus enhancing the integrated systemic intent of this chapter, the integration of EMDR, which is a psychotherapeutic and neurobiological protocol, with a family systems model such as the Metaframeworks Perspective, in healing psychological trauma in an external family system such as the couple subsystem.

In his 2010 book *The Mindful Therapist*, Siegel specifies,

> Presence permits us to be open to others, and to ourselves. Attunement is the act of focusing on another person (or ourselves) to bring into our awareness the internal state of the other into interpersonal attunement (or the self, in intrapersonal attunement). Resonance is the coupling of two autonomous entities into a functional whole. A and B are in resonance as each attunes to the other, and both are changed as they take the internal state of one another into themselves. When such resonance is enacted in a positive regard, a deep feeling of coherence emerges with the subjective sensation of harmony. When two strings of an instrument resonate, for example, each is changed by the impact of the other. Naturally, as A is changed because of B, B is then changed further as A's changes induce further changes in B. Two literally become linked as one. The whole is larger than the sum of the individual parts. In many ways we feel 'close' or 'heard' or 'seen' by another person when we can detect that he has attuned

to us and taken us inside of his own mind. When we ourselves register this attunement, either consciously or not, our own state can change. The observed takes in the observer having taken her in, and the two become joined. This is resonance.

(p. 54)

Siegel's further elaborations on resonance take us back to the therapeutic process and the role of therapist discussed in Chapter 3, adding yet another dimension:

We come to the relational role of being a guide, perhaps, or a teacher, and in some ways an attachment figure—someone who provides a safe haven where the other can be deeply seen and feel safe and secure. At other times we are the expert on the mind, and perhaps on the brain and relationships too, and on the notion of health and unhealth, ease and disease. Yet our patients are also experts in their own right, deeply knowledgeable in other domains. Our patients are certainly expert in being themselves. No one else shares this distinctive skill base. Even without self-awareness, the people who are our clients are still the 'best' them that they can be. So we come as individuals, each with our own expertise, to find one another in this journey across time. Our job is not to be one who knows everything, but the one who is present, attuned and open for resonance with what is.

(p. 56)

In the end, Siegel's mindful conceptualizations parallel my efforts to advance the integration of EMDR and the Metaframeworks perspective in healing psychological trauma within the systems paradigm. Indeed, mindfulness practice puts the icing on the proverbial cake, in this case, the integrative cake: it integrates and centers the traumatized psyche, which is of course the goal of integrated therapeutic practice.

References

Bardin, A. (2004). "EMDR within a Family Systems Perspective." *Journal of Family Psychotherapy, 51* (3), 47–61.

Bateson, G. (1972). *Steps to an Ecology of Mind.* New York: Ballantine.

Breunlin, D., Schwartz, R.C., & Mac Kune-Karrer, B. (1992). *Metaframeworks: Transcending the Models of Family Therapy.* San Francisco: Jossey-Bass Publishers.

Breunlin, D. (1999). "Toward a Theory of Constraints." (2nd ed) *Journal of Marital and Family Therapy, 25* (1), 365–382.

Cook, A., Blaustein, M., Spinazzola, J., & van der Kolk. (2003). "Complex Trauma in Children and Adolescents: White Paper from the National Child Trauma Stress Network Complex Trauma Task Force." *The National Child Traumatic Stress Network (NCTSN).* www.nctsnet.org/nctsn_assets/pdfs/edu_materials/ CouplesTrauma_all.pdf Accessed September 16, 2016

Herbine-Blank, T. (2013). "Self in Relationship: An Introduction to IFS Therapy." Edited by E.L. Ziskind & M. Sweezy. *Internal Family Systems Therapy: New Dimensions.* (pp. 55–71). New York: Routledge: Taylor & Francis Group.

Johnson, L., & Moore, M. (2017). "EMDR with Couples and Families: Integrating EMDR Therapy with Relationship Enhancement Therapy." *International Family Therapy Association Conference.* Malaga, Spain. March 15–18, 2017.

Johnson, S.M., & Williams-Keeler, L. (1998). "Creating Healing Relationships for Couples Dealing with Trauma: The use of Emotionally Focused Marital Therapy." *Journal of Marital and Family Therapy, 24* (1), 25–40.

Kaslow, F.W., Nurse, A.R., & Thompson, P. (Eds). (2002). "EMDR in Conjuction with Family Systems." *EMDR as an Integrative Psychotherapy Approach.* (pp. 289–318). Washington, DC: American Psychological Association.

Maxfield, L., Kaslow, F.W., & Shapiro, F. (Eds). (2007). "The Integration of EMDR and Family Systems Therapy." *Handbook of EMDR and Family Therapy Processes.* (pp. 407–421). Hoboken, NJ: John Wiley & Sons.

Moses, M.D. (Ed). (2007). "Enhancing Attachments: Conjoint Couple Therapy." *Handbook of EMDR and Family Therapy Processes.* (pp. 146–168). Hoboken, NJ: John Wiley & Sons.

Pinsof, W.M. (1995). *Integrative Problem-Centered Therapy: A Synthesis of Family, Individual, and Biological Therapies.* New York: BasicBooks, A Subsidiary of Perseus Books.

Schwartz, R.C. (1997). *Internal Family Systems.* New York: The Guilford Press.

Shapiro, F. (2001). *Eye Movement Desensitization and Reprocessing: Basic Principles, Protocols, and Procedures.* New York: The Guilford Press.

Shapiro, F., & Kaslow, F.W. (Eds). (2007). "Preface." *Handbook of EMDR and Family Therapy Processes* (pp. xxi–xxiii). Hoboken, NJ: John Wiley & Sons.

Siegel, D.J. (Ed). (2007). "Forward." *Handbook of EMDR and Family Therapy Processes* (pp. xiii–xx). Hoboken, NJ: John Wiley & Sons.

Siegel, D.J. (2010). *The Mindful Therapist: A Clinician's Guide to Mindsight and Neural Integration.* New York and London: W.W. Norton and Company.

Smythe, N.J., & Poole, D. (2002). "EMDR and Cognitive-Behavioral Therapy: Exploring Convergence and Divergence." In Shapiro, F. (Ed.), *EMDR as an Integrative Psychotherapy Approach: Experts of Diverse Orientations Explore the Paradigm Prism* (pp. 151–180). Washington, DC: American Psychological Association.

Sweezy, M., & Ziskind, E.L. (Eds.) (2013). *Internal Family Systems: New Dimensions* (Ed). (2013). New York: Routledge: Taylor & Francis Group.

van der Kolk, B. (2014). *The Body Keeps the Score: Brain, Mind, and Body in the Healing of Trauma.* New York: Viking.

Wesselmann, D. (Ed). (2007). "Treating Attachment Issues through EMDR and a Family Systems Approach." *Handbook of EMDR and Family Therapy Processes* (pp. 95–112). Hoboken, NJ: John Wiley & Sons.

6 Summary, Clinical Implications and Further Research

In his 2015 book *Trauma and Memory: Brain and Body in a Search for the Living Past*, Peter A. Levine observes:

> When we are able to 'look back' at a traumatic memory from an empowered stance, the recollection will be updated as though this agency had been available and fully functional at the time of the original trauma. This newly reconsolidated experience then becomes the new updated memory where the (empowered) present somatic experience profoundly alters the (past) memory. *These emerging resources become the bridging of past and present—'the remembered present.'* This memory updating in no way takes away from the truth that a particularly traumatizing event really did happen, that it caused egregious harm, and that grief and outrage may be significant components to restoring dignity and a deep honoring of the Self. From this present-based platform of self-compassion, the memories can be gradually softened, reshaped and rewoven into the fabric of one's identity.
>
> (p. 142)

Given my background and personal and professional journey (see Preface), the analogy that Levine offers next resonates with both the process of treating those suffering from psychological trauma and my fervent expectations for all those *lost in translation*. As Levine expresses it,

> This brings to mind the ancient Japanese tradition of repairing broken porcelain antiquities by reuniting the fragments with seams of gold. The repair of the shattered pieces renders exquisitely transformed works of art, just as healing the wounds of trauma gives rise to the natural world of ebb and flow, where empowerment, harmony, self-compassion, and dignity are restored. What could be more beautiful and more valuable?
>
> (p. 143)

Yes, indeed, what could be more beautiful!

The present chapter has several goals, namely, to briefly summarize the essence of my previous chapters, to make clear the clinical implications of their content, to highlight the importance of entry-level trauma education for future practitioners, to underline the need for future evidence-based research, and to indicate what this research should look like. My hope is that I have provided fellow researchers and clinicians with an *integrated* approach for healing psychological trauma in family systems and have inspired them to continue my passionate journey.

Summary

The purpose of my Preface was to help other clinicians in re-thinking their own professional narratives in order to help those suffering from trauma as well as to reconsider their own professional practices in an effort to empower them to constantly seek to improve their therapeutic skills and to continue their quest for knowledge. I also hope that I provided some relief to other clinicians who might have witnessed their own psychological trauma and inspire them to use their experiences to better understand and identify with the healing process of their clients.

My Introduction outlined the premise of this book and briefly explained the rationale of the subsequent chapters to support my inclusive and postmodern clinical endeavor. First and foremost, however, I addressed the importance of understanding the language and etiology of trauma and its primary place in the vast majority of mental health diagnoses. I also explained my rationale for including the visual presence of the *integrated* sacred space of a mandala, intended to help clinicians understand visually how the premise of my book would unfold.

In Chapter 1, "A World of Trauma," I set the stage through language, etiology, and statistics. With this in mind, I reiterated the prevalence of diverse and horrifying trauma statistics and the fact that psychological trauma still remains under-recognized, under-diagnosed, and under-treated on many clinical levels. In this chapter, I also addressed the etymology of "trauma," and the severity of the impact of multidimensional inter-personal fragmentation, i.e., the extreme fragmentation of self-structure that occurs in the traumatized brain, body, and psyche. Specifically, I indicated how overwhelming emotions can interfere with proper memory processing, cognitive processing, and somatic functioning, and how the vast majority of mental health diagnoses are rooted in previous traumas. It was particularly surprising for this author to have grasped the notion that many of the concepts mentioned above were already being addressed by Pierre Janet in 1889 in his work *L'automatisme psychologique*. I found myself asking why it took so long for his theories and concepts to be actualized in a *world of trauma*.

I selected a visual integrated counterpart, the mandala, to introduce my readers to what a holistic and integrated approach, with EMDR as the centerpiece, might look like, one that would continue to be addressed throughout my book. With the advent of a society experiencing heightened terror, apathy, and confusion, the need to re-think more *integrated* approaches was advocated for all clinicians and researchers. The Sandy Hook school shooting, which took place only a few miles from where I work, served as an example. We are only now beginning to hear some of the victims' painful narratives. I found myself asking the question "Why is it, that only now, almost six years later, this population is healing, i.e., achieving the ability to free themselves from insecure attachment issues; to re-integrate the Self; to understand the basis of their emotions and cognitions; to self-regulate; to feel safe to reprocess the toxic traumatic memories; and to heal from their trauma in order to connect, communicate, and regain equity and intimacy both in the internal and external systems paradigm?"

In Chapter 2, I set my sights on exploring another crucial topic, a set of possible quagmires (i.e., the inefficacy of the DSM-V, the fact that medication was not healing pervasive trauma, and why talk therapy alone did not seem to work) in an attempt to understand why the prevalence of psychological trauma as discussed in Chapter 1 continued. While I realized that each of the familiar tools applied to trauma, from medication to talk therapy, offered a great deal, they all fell short when it came to healing traumatic memories and experiences in their totality.

The next chapter focused on the neurobiological Eye Movement Desensitization and Reprocessing (EMDR) psychotherapeutic and neurobiological protocol developed by Francine Shapiro. Much attention was given to the endorsement of EMDR by an impressive list of scholars, researchers, practitioners, and government and private agencies. The core concepts of EMDR were detailed including the Adaptive Information Processing (AIP) model, the eight-phase modality, the three-pronged approach to healing trauma, and the role of the EMDR therapist. Regarding the last, I addressed the complexities surrounding the effects of trauma that could also affect how clients present within the therapeutic milieu, which could confuse inexperienced therapists and get them "stuck." I considered, for example, how if they are not careful, therapists might engage in treatment without ever hearing their clients' struggles with trauma, which many times might be directly related to their presenting problems (e.g., depression, anxiety, social isolation, marital conflict, and a variety of other diagnoses). I also reviewed selected evidence-based studies that bolstered the power of EMDR in healing psychological trauma. Finally, I researched other trauma-based neurobiological therapies in an effort to maintain the objectivity of my support of EMDR as the first line of treatment for healing psychological trauma within a systems frame.

In Chapter 4, I focused on how to enhance the EMDR protocol as an *integrated* approach by discussing a diverse number of effective pre-EMDR practices. I offered the benefits of providing psychoeducation to our clients, researching and utilizing the most evidence-based diverse screening and diagnostic tools such as sophisticated intake reports, self-report assessments, standardized psychometric tools, clinical interviews, and the genogram. I lobbied for the assessment of attachment styles and the exploration of their neurophysiological foundations as proposed in the polyvagal theory and explored how one might alter insecure attachment styles impacting communication patterns, relational contexts, and dysfunctional behaviors. This chapter also considered the importance of working through the Internal Family Systems (IFS) model in an effort to lower the extremity of *parts* and promote Self leadership as well as the importance of mindfulness, including both its theoretical and practical aspects and its consonance with neuroplasticity. Both were discussed with the intent of enhancing safety, self-regulation, and attending to the somatic and spiritual "Self" of those suffering from psychological trauma. My thesis was that all of these modalities and cutting-edge research strengthen the preparation phase in EMDR. The heart of Chapter 5 was the attempt to view the unique integration of Shapiros' eight-phase EMDR trauma protocol and a sophisticated and inclusive Family Systems Therapy (FST) modality, namely the Metaframeworks perspective, through the lens of a couple suffering from psychological trauma.

Clinical Implications

I strived to make it transparent for my readers, from my clinical experiences and research, that trauma affects individuals and couples in multifaceted and multimodal ways and that all aspects of their lives are impacted. Trauma affects the cognitive and physical ability of my clients, their mood, intimate relationships, and work performance/relationships. Therefore, I hypothesized a persistent need for trauma treatment that utilizes multilevel and multidimensional diagnostic processes and the integration of multiple treatment modalities that can address the full range of trauma symptomology. In my practice, I discovered significant improvement in my population suffering from psychological trauma (e.g., unstable mood symptoms, reactivity, somatic complaints) when utilizing an *integrated* approach, namely, an *integrated* neurobiological protocol such as EMDR with an equally *integrated* Family Systems Therapy (FST) modality such as the Metaframeworks perspective. As I hope my readers have witnessed, this approach proved most effective due to the latter modality's ability to quickly and effectively assess and treat the complexities of the human condition in particular populations with complex clinical presentations like those which arise from psychological trauma.

Preparing Future Practitioners

I would now like to bring to the attention of my readers the need to address psychological trauma in MFT practice, primarily the education of our students who will most certainly encounter individuals, couples, and family systems experiencing traumatic events in their clinical practice. While we train our students in systems theories to treat a wide range of mental health diagnoses, there remains a fracture in preparing them to face the complexities within the trauma paradigm. Erica J. W. Kanewischer, however, recognizes the inherent need to prepare our future clinicians at the entry level. Teaching in family studies at the undergraduate level, Kanewischer recognizes the benefits of incorporating trauma education for her students who typically "go on to pursue graduate education in MFT." She designed a senior seminar course at Saint Olaf College in Northfield, Minnesota, titled "Families and Trauma." Her course objectives include understanding the symptoms of psychological trauma and accompanying attachment issues, how to cultivate empathy for individuals and their families suffering from psychological trauma, understanding their personal experiences of trauma, understanding the attachment styles and intergenerational trauma within the frame of those suffering from psychological trauma, and how to create an environment of safety, while paying attention to the all-important cultural and spiritual resources and resiliency factors that are brought to the therapeutic space (Kanewischer, 2017). In the mind of this author and, I hope, in the minds of my readers, it is essential to educate our MFT students to begin to face the specter of trauma at the entry level of their studies and to continue rigorous "trauma" training throughout their subsequent graduate studies in an effort to heal psychological trauma within the systems paradigm.

Future Research

Generally speaking, we can envision a unified research arc for the continued investigation of EMDR, an arc that has four components. We already have the first component: there are a host of careful studies that confirm that EMDR is more effective than placebo in the treatment of the effects of psychological trauma.

Second, it is desirable to have research that teases out what it is that is uniquely effective in EMDR. There are strong reasons to suppose that the bilateral stimulation at the heart of EMDR therapy is crucial, but, ideally, future research will demonstrate that the key to EMDR's efficacy is indeed bilateral stimulation, and not simply the sort of confrontation with one's trauma that EMDR shares with an approach such as Cognitive Behavioral Therapy.

Third, for any treatment modality to have scientific validity, we must have hypotheses that propose specific neurological mechanisms of action at work in that treatment (e.g., neuroplasticity and the polyvagal theory). As I have already indicated, such hypotheses already exist where EMDR is concerned. They include the contention that EMDR taps into some of the mechanisms of REM sleep.

Finally, we must hope that theorists can produce testable predictions based on their hypotheses. It is only then that we will be able to move into the laboratory and either falsify specific hypotheses or provide them significant empirical support. This is an ambitious goal, one that will require significant amounts of time and resources to accomplish, but it is the natural endpoint of the research arc.

On a more detailed, specific level, I offer the following nine considerations that can help guide future research.

1. In their 2005 study "Posttraumatic Stress Disorder Treatment Outcome Research: The Study of Unrepresentative Samples," Joseph Spinazzola, Margaret Blaustein, and Bessel A. van der Kolk provide us with one of many vital openings for future research:

    > Findings reveal that many published reports omitted vital data including exclusion criteria and rates, demographics, and trauma exposure therapy. Moreover severe comorbid psychopathology, a common feature of treatment-seeking individuals with PTSD, emerged as the predominant reason for exclusion across studies. Subsequently published studies exhibited improved reporting of sample characteristics and demonstrated comparable outcomes despite inclusion of more diverse trauma exposure samples. Findings indicate the need for future efficacy research to adopt more comprehensive reporting requirements and to test the applicability of validated treatments to individuals suffering from as yet unstudied combinations of PTSD and prevalent comorbid disorders.
    >
    > (p. 425)

    As I indicated briefly in my Introduction, there exist a multitude of mental health diagnoses that are co-morbid with PTSD. This is substantiated by Spinazzola et al. when they point out that "the convergence of leading epidemiological data clearly indicates that PTSD rarely occurs alone, and has routine comorbidity rates of 80%" (p. 426). Furthermore, regarding the omission of demographics, the authors recognize that "demographic and baseline severity characteristics of dropouts are not consistently included in the results of treatment outcome studies" (p. 427).

2. There is also an inherent need for evidence-based practice as well as evidence-based research. Evidence-based practice involves curious, creative, and thoughtful decision-making. It offers the best available research evidence centered on whether and why a treatment works as well as clinical expertise in order to quickly locate each patient's unique diagnoses, along with the risks and benefits of potential intervention and clients' preferences and values (see Berke et al. (2011). The Metaframeworks model's assumption of *perspectivism* coheres with the need for curious, creative, and thoughtful decision-making, since *perspectivism* implies that we can never know a complete reality. As such, we must continually shift our care regarding diagnoses, hypothesis, and interventions.

3. We need both responsible qualitative and quantitative research. Qualitative research is based on trends and discussions and open-ended interviews in an effort to gather data to identify major themes, while quantitative research gathers data in a way that can be put in numerical form and allows for statistical analysis.

4. Ongoing investigations of the integrated approach I am proposing also need to utilize randomized controlled studies with large samples that demonstrate reliability or consistency of results and validity (i.e., measuring what they were intended to measure). It is also desirable to carry out longitudinal quantitative outcome studies to support the efficacy of integrating the EMDR neurobiological protocol with Family Systems Therapy (FST) modalities such as the Metaframeworks perspective.
5. Inherently stronger research will also come from analyzing two trauma treatments and paying careful attention to the base-line scores and drop-out rates when working with two modalities. This became clear to me when I taught a university graduate research course in Marriage and Family Therapy (MFT), as did the fact that two or more randomized controlled outcome studies was highly advised in order to determine the significant strengths of one study. In addition, when small or weak studies occurred, I advocated that my students recognize that a statistical meta-analysis (i.e., statistical methods for combining the results of two or more studies), although beyond the purview of this book, was necessary to coordinate results in the hopes of drawing a stronger conclusion (see Patten, 2007).
6. Future EMDR research in general must continue to improve not only in taking into account clients' background characteristics, demographics, and the prevalence of PTSD with comorbid disorders, but also needs to improve the type of diagnostic tools (e.g., self-report, clinical interviews, and standardized psychometric instruments) addressed in Chapter 4. That research must help us diagnose the client's ability to self-regulate and socialize and to assess complex trauma with specific case conceptualization. By implementing diagnostic tools, we can quickly locate target symptoms and evaluate psychological trauma from start to finish.
7. Future research should also attend to variables of time, beginning with the time of the traumatic experience, and the frequency and severity of the traumatic experiences (indicated by the symptom cluster), and continuing with long-term follow-up and outcome measurements.
8. There is also a special need for continued and responsible consideration of racially, ethnically, culturally, and gender-diverse evidence-based research. This is a fundamental ethical responsibility. And we must continue to address clinical ethical considerations: asking questions of our therapists, for example, such as, "Where can the therapist get stuck?" "Is the therapist attuned with her parts?" and "Is the Self of the therapist getting in the way?"—all critical in the maintenance of ethical practices.
9. We must take into consideration the fact that when working with individuals traumatized by terrorist attacks, environmental disasters, and other forms of community violence, researching trauma becomes more problematic since post-disaster intervention by first-aid responders, forensic specialists, local authorities, and government agencies weakens studies that utilize controlled groups rather than an analogue wait list, as discussed in Chapter 3.

In the end, it has become apparent to me that our profession needs to be practiced in a responsible, creative, and curious way by appropriately trained individuals holding to the highest ethical standards. As such, it is of the utmost importance to consult the International Practice Guidelines for Post-trauma Mental Health (ISTSS), which is frequently updated to provide the best of care to those suffering from trauma. I hope for myself and my colleagues the continual giving of what is the best in ourselves in order to enable those with traumatic experiences to attain peace in their lives and genuinely to flourish.

References

Berke, D.M., Rozell, C.A., Hogan, T.O., Norcross, J.A., & Karpiak, C.P. (April 2011). "What Clinical Psychologists Know about Evidence-Based Practice: Familiarity with Online Resources and Research Methods." *Journal of Clinical Psychology, 67* (4), 329–339.

Kanewischer, E.J.W. (2017). "Teaching Trauma from a Systemic Perspective." *Family Therapy Magazine (ftm), 16* (1), 36–39.

Levine, P.A. (2015). *Trauma and Memory: Brain and Body in a Search for the Living Past*. Berkeley, CA: North Atlantic Books.

Patten, M.L. (2007). *Understanding Research Methods* (6th ed.). Los Angeles: Pyrczak Publishing.

Spinazzola, J., Blaustein, M., van der Kolk, B.A. (2005). "Posttraumatic Stress Disorder Treatment Outcome Research: The Study of Unrepresentative Samples." *Journal of Traumatic Stress, 18* (5), 425–436.

Appendices

Appendix 1
Not All the Victims Die

There it is again. The headline: "Shooting at Ft Lauderdale Airport: 5 Dead." Just another day in the U.S.A.

Mass shootings are becoming a common occurrence in this country. And for most people outside the affected communities, the process becomes routine: they see the photos of the victims, express outrage, maybe shed a tear, and even say a prayer. And then it's over. Turn the page and go back to business as usual. But there is one thing that they cannot glean from the photos of the murdered: in a mass shooting, not all of the victims die.

I am a victim of a mass shooting, a gun violence survivor. I was in the same hallway as those who were massacred at Sandy Hook Elementary School on December 14, 2012. I heard every gunshot. I heard the terrified screams of 6- and 7-year-olds, in stereo, outside my room and over the loudspeaker. Then I heard the deafening silence when the screaming stopped, as I hid in a small, dark bathroom with a little boy who asked me, "Mrs. Wilk, where's Superman?"

Superman didn't come, and now that little boy is, like so many others, a victim of a mass shooting. We were fortunate enough to survive. Our families did not lose us. But we had to walk that hallway, stepping through the drops of blood staining the floor of our elementary school. We walked past the lifeless bodies of our principal and school psychologist. We heard the sounds of the glass crunching beneath our feet, the glass from the windows that the madman shot out to get into our beautiful little school. We survived, physically uninjured, mentally raped.

Parts of the story are often the same, a troubled person, usually male, often young and white, targets the unsuspecting and innocent. He is either mentally unstable or just plain angry. And he is in possession of large-capacity firearms. It's amazing how much damage one lone madman with an arsenal can do to a community.

It's a ripple effect. In the center, of course, are the dead. In our case—20 first graders and 6 educators. Lives full of promise, snuffed out in a matter of minutes, in the most terrifying way. **Senseless. Violent. Tragic**. These are the first victims of the Sandy Hook shooting. But beyond these victims, there are so many more. Their families, parents, siblings, children are left to navigate life without their loved one; left to try to make sense of the loss. How do you move forward? How do you learn to live with the loss of someone you love so deeply, when the circumstance is so horrific and surreal? How do you get beyond the grief and anger? I don't pretend to understand their struggles. I cannot begin to comprehend the depth of their pain.

Beyond the families, and often seen as a mere "footnote" in the story, are those who witnessed the shootings. In Ft. Lauderdale, an airport terminal full of travelers and staff. In Orlando, a nightclub full of party goers. At Sandy Hook, an entire school full of children, ages 5–10.

There are the first-grade survivors who actually SAW THEIR TEACHERS and FRIENDS GUNNED DOWN! A few were able to escape the room and run from the school when the shooter stopped to reload. Others hid and were lucky that the shooter took his own life before he searched any further. Little children, covered in the blood of their friends and their teachers. Stories of these last few years would break your heart, as these small survivors try to come to terms with what they have seen. From the child who is terrified of dark clouds passing overhead, to the one who thought Santa Claus had placed him on the "naughty" list because he was part of something so evil. These children will likely need mental health services for the rest of their lives. And yet, they are not counted among the victims.

There were second and third graders in that hallway as well. They walked the same path my little friend and I walked, heard and saw what we did. The entire school heard the gunshots and screams over the intercom. The report of an AR-15 sounds an awful lot like pounding hammers or metal chairs toppling, as it echoes thru elementary school hallways. Pop! Pop! Pop! You would be amazed to learn how many normal, everyday things sound like an AR-15 in the halls of an elementary school. Life will never be the same for these kids.

Then there is the surviving staff. Some were physically injured; others tended to the injured, knowing the gunman was just outside the door; some even heard the words the gunman yelled as he took the lives of those precious souls; and others were treated as criminals and left vulnerable in the heat of the madness. All are left with sounds and images of horror engrained in our psyches. We were the untrained first responders, doing everything we could to keep our charges safe. Yet we are not considered victims.

All of the staff of December 2012, whether present that morning or not, suffer greatly. We live with the memories of the days that followed the 14th. We had so many wakes and funerals to attend, one spouse created a spreadsheet to help us decide which services we could manage. Imagine attending the funeral of a first grader, then doing it again an hour later, and again the next day and the next. Then having to go back to a school without our leadership, without some teachers, without an entire class and a half of sweet, innocent first graders, feeling the void with the darkest understanding of why, yet still not comprehending it.

We lost our school and were moved to a school in a neighboring town. It was a comfort to be together, yet each morning, the drive down that long driveway was a painful reminder. Every day my heart felt like it would rip from of my chest as I entered the property. But we had a school full of children who needed us. So we went. Day after day, week after week, month after month, walking the halls in a daze, finding little corners where the children couldn't see us break down. And break down we did, over and over. We still do, but we've gotten really good at pretending everything is OK. Of course, that was the directive from the beginning. But that is another story.

Sometimes it feels like the world thinks we weren't even there. Concern is expressed for the families, the first responders, and "the community," as it should be. But rarely over the years has there been concern shown for the staff or the children who were in the building that day. This lack of acknowledgement is dismissive and hurtful. It's as if people believe that since we were showing up every day, we were "fine." Well, we weren't fine then and some of us are only just getting the necessary treatment now.

With all these survivors comes a whole other set of victims: their loved ones. It is hard to fathom the difficulty of watching someone you love with all your heart, suffer the aftermath of a mass shooting. You hold up the crumbling mass, take care of the day to day while she/he is curled in the fetal position afraid to move. You watch the life you had together fade into darkness; not knowing if your family will ever be happy again. Will your loved one ever lose that far-away look and regain that "love of life" that had been so vibrant? Your family is a victim of a mass shooting.

Though it is true that police are trained for emergency situations, no one could ever have enough training to shield them from the horrors they faced on 12/14. No amount of training could protect the firefighters and EMTs. Nothing could prepare the hospital staff that waited and waited, just to find that there were so few coming that could be treated. Even first responders are victims.

Grandparents, aunts, uncles, cousins, neighbors, clergy, and funeral directors are victims. School bus drivers, friends, former students, classmates, teammates, and all of their families are victims. Parents who had to put their little ones on a school bus days after the massacre and pretend that everything was fine are victims. Then went home to cry and pray for their children's safe return . . . FROM SCHOOL! Staff at other schools who had to welcome those children like everything was fine. Even others with no direct connection to the school, who lost their sense of security and had their innocence shattered in a matter of minutes. The list goes on and on of all the victims who continue to suffer.

Our little town is trying to get back to a place where the first day of school is something to celebrate. We are trying to find ways to stop the dread that comes with the approach of Christmas, because it means we will have to face yet another "anniversary." We are trying to learn to live with the "new normal" that will never be truly normal again. The effects of mass murder do not go away after the last funeral has ended. They linger on for years. Just ask the folks from Columbine, Virginia Tech, Fort Hood, Red Lake, Seal Beach, Nickel Mines, and countless others.

Now, as I read the headlines of each new event, it is 12/14 all over again. I once again hear the screams. I think of the new members of the "Survivors Club." I think of the traumatized, who will forever jump at every noise. I think of the families who will never fill the void left behind. And I ask you to please, remember the victims. *All of the victims.* Mourn for the fallen, but remember, for every person who dies, there are many, many more that survive and have to live with the aftermath.

Karen Wilk, former Para-Educator at the Sandy Hook Elementary School in Sandy Hook, Connecticut, is a Neurofeedback Technician at the Neurovation Center in Sandy Hook, Connecticut. She is a talented writer and a Sandy Hook Survivor.

Appendix 2
Overview of Eight Phases of EMDR Treatment

Phase	*Purpose*	*Procedures*
Phase 1 Client History	• Obtain background information • Identify suitability for EMDR treatment • Identify processing targets from positive and negative events in client's life	• Administer standard history-taking questionnaires and diagnostic psychometrics • Review of criteria and resources • Ask questions regarding (1) past events that have laid the ground-work for the pathology, (2) current triggers, and (3) future needs
Phase 2 Preparation	• Prepare appropriate clients for EMDR processing of targets • Stabilize and increase access to positive affects: (Calm/Safe Place)	• Educate regarding the symptom picture • Teach metaphors and techniques that foster stabilization and a sense of personal self-mastery and control
Phase 3 Assessment	• Access the target for EMDR processing by stimulating primary aspects of the memory	• Elicit the image, negative belief currently held, desired positive belief, current emotion, and physical sensation and baseline measures
Phase 4 Desensitization	• Process experiences toward an adaptive resolution (0 SUD level) • Fully process all channels to allow a complete assimilation of memories • Incorporate templates for positive experiences	• Use standardized EMDR protocols allowing the spontaneous emergence of insights, emotions, physical sensations, and other memories • Use "Cognitive Interweave" to open blocked processing by elicitation of more adaptive information

(*Continued*)

Phase	Purpose	Procedures
Phase 5 Installation	• Increase connection to positive cognitive networks • Increase generalization effects within associated memories	• Identify the best positive cognition (initial or emergent) • Enhance the validity of the desired positive belief to a 7 VOC
Phase 6 Body Scan	• Complete processing of any residual disturbance associated with the target	• Concentration on and processing of any residual physical sensations
Phase 7 Closure	• Ensure client stability at the completion of an EMDR session and between sessions	• Use of guided imagery or self control techniques if needed • Brief regarding expectations and behavioral reports between sessions
Phase 8 Reevaluation	• Evaluation of treatment effects • Ensure comprehensive processing over time	• Explore what has emerged since last session • Access memory from last session • Evaluation of integration within larger social system

Francine Shapiro (2012), The EMDR Approach to Psychotherapy.

EMDR Institute: Basic Training Course, Part II of The Two Part Basic Training, p. 6, EMDR Institute [Reprinted with permission]

Appendix 3
Negative and Positive Cognitions

Negative Cognitions	Positive Cognitions
Responsibility/Defectiveness	
I'm not good enough	I am good enough/fine as I am
I don't deserve love	I deserve love; I can have love
I am a bad person	I am a good (loving) person
I am incompetent	I am competent
I am worthless/inadequate	I am worthy; I am worthwhile
I am shameful	I am honorable
I am not loveable	I am loveable
I deserve only bad things	I deserve good things
I am permanently damaged	I am/can be healthy
I am ugly/my body is hateful	I am fine/attractive/loveable
I do not deserve . . .	I can have/deserve . . .
I am stupid/not smart enough	I am intelligent/able to learn
I am insignificant/unimportant	I am significant/important
I am a disappointment	I am OK just the way I am
I deserve to die	I deserve to live
I deserve to be miserable	I deserve to be happy
I am different/don't belong	I am OK as I am
I have to be perfect (out of inadequacy)	I am fine the way I am
Responsibility: Action	
I should have done something*	I did the best I could
I did something wrong*	I learned/can learn from it
I should have known better*	I do the best I can/I can learn
*What does this say about you? (e.g., therefore I am . . .)	
I am shameful/I am stupid/I am a bad person	I'm fine as I am
I am inadequate/weak	I am adequate/strong

Safety/Vulnerability

I cannot trust anyone	I can choose whom to trust
I cannot protect myself	I can learn to protect myself
I am in danger	It's over; I am safe now
I am not safe	I am safe now
I am going to die	I am safe now
It's not OK (safe) to feel/show my emotions	I can safely feel/show my emotions

Power/Control

I am not in control	I am now in control
I am powerless/helpless	I now have choices
I cannot get what I want	I can get what I want
I cannot stand up for myself	I can make my needs known
I cannot let it out	I can choose to let it out
I cannot be trusted	I can be trusted
I cannot trust myself	I can/learn to trust myself
I cannot trust my judgement	I can trust my judgement
I am a failure/will fail	I can succeed
I cannot succeed	I can succeed
I have to be perfect/please everyone	I can be myself/make mistakes
I can't handle it (I'm out of control)	I can handle it

Francine Shapiro (2012), The EMDR Approach to Psychotherapy.

EMDR Institute; Basic Training Course, Part II of The Two Part Basic Training, p. 9, EMDR Institute [Reprinted with permission]

Appendix 4
The Role of Neurofeedback

The field of mental health is on the verge of change. This comment is in no way a criticism of the efforts and intent of those of us who labor in the field using talk therapy or medication to treat; rather, such change should be expected in the face of growing demand for services, intensified research seeking empirically verifiable models, and the dynamic expansion of the neurosciences. Moreover, this change is arguably necessary, given the current climate of dissatisfaction with diagnostic processes and the DSM-V as an accurate and effective means of describing mental health issues. Change, in this case, means more treatment options, better diagnostic processes, and better outcomes. At the forefront of this change is a growing awareness that the application of neuroscience to the mental health field will transform the way we think about, diagnose, and treat the organ that is primarily responsible for human behavior.

This paradigm shift in mental health is of particular importance in the treatment of trauma-related disorders. Post-traumatic stress disorder (PTSD) has arguably stronger physiological underpinnings than any other mental health disorder. The hallmark symptoms of PTSD are a manifestation of the body's biological reaction to traumatic experiences. The literature on the physiological effects of trauma is vast and provides irrefutable evidence of the alterations that are associated with PTSD. Replicated evidence of increased sympathetic nervous system dominance has been found in individuals with PTSD including decreased heart rate variability, increased heart rate, and increased blood pressure (Pole, 2007). Numerous neuro-imaging studies have also shown hypo-activations in the prefrontal cortex, anterior cingulate cortex, and thalamus in individuals with PTSD compared to control groups (Etkin and Wagner, 2007). These regions of the brain are involved in the experience of emotions, emotional regulation, and the regulation of fear extinction. Additional neuroimaging studies have found altered functioning in three important brain networks in individuals with PTSD: the central executive network (CEN), salience network (SN), and default mode network (DMN) (Lanius et al., 2015). Each network dysfunction is thought to be associated with specific clinical PTSD symptoms including cognitive dysfunction, hyper-arousal, and an altered sense of self. It is for this reason that treatment modalities used to treat trauma must be able to resolve the physiological alterations associated with trauma just as much as or more than the psychological distress.

As awareness of the need for effective trauma treatments has grown, EMDR and neurofeedback have emerged as two promising modalities that seek to meet this need. Both of these treatment approaches have been rapidly growing in popularity and efficacy in the treatment of trauma due to their ability to produce change through neuro-biological mechanisms—EMDR utilizes bilateral stimulation and mindfulness techniques while neurofeedback utilizes operant conditioning of brain activity. Although EMDR and neurofeedback are markedly different in their approaches, they share the abilities of reducing physiological arousal and enabling individuals to process and re-integrate traumatic memories. In our clinical experience, these modalities can be used simultaneously and complementarily to expedite therapeutic progress.

Neurofeedback, also referred to as EEG biofeedback, is a non-invasive, safe, and enduring treatment that focuses on the remediation of symptoms associated with mental health disorders. It involves the application of behavioral (or more specifically, neuronal) conditioning through the regulation of electrical patterns in the brain. Neurofeedback treatment sets up a brain-computer interface wherein the individual is rewarded or inhibited with audible and/or visual cues according to parameters set by the clinician. At The Neurovation Center, we do this while the patient watches a movie. When a patient's brain regulates its electrical patterns within normative ranges, they are rewarded by having a bright image on the TV screen and/or receiving an added audible cue. When they drop below an established performance set-point, the system dims the screen and/or arrests the audible cue. The human brain, intuitively attuned to associating patterns with rewards, automatically and pre-consciously adapts its own neuro-electrical processes in order to watch the movie. This is the feedback loop for which neurofeedback is named. As the brain receives feedback via rewards, it learns to adjust its own neuro-electrical patterns.

Why might this shift in neuro-electrical patterns be so important, and what makes neurofeedback an effective and viable treatment for mental health disorders? To answer, we note that the central nervous system, like all systems in the body, functions best if within certain measurable ranges. We take this for granted with other systems, such as when a person has headaches because of high blood pressure in the circulatory system. Return blood pressure to normal ranges and the headache simply goes away. It is, interestingly, something of a novel idea in the mental health field to extend this principle to the electrical activity of the brain. It is now clear, though, that behavioral symptoms (for instance, rumination, hyperactivity, lack of motivation, mood instability, etc.) are likely to arise when neuro-electrical patterns fall outside of those norms. Assessment and treatment for neurofeedback uses EEG (electroencephalogram) technology, routinely employed by the medical field as a valid and reliable analytical tool. With the EEG, we can measure a number of electrical features of brave waves such as frequency, amplitude, and phase relationships (amongst many others). When measurements fall outside of normative ranges or present as atypical, we can correlate the nature and anatomical location of the dysregulation with expressed symptomology. Simply stated, we can now actually see the symptoms associated with mental health diagnoses such as anxiety, ADHD, depression, OCD, and PTSD in the baseline electrical rhythms of an individual's EEG. Change those patterns and you can remediate symptoms.

An important caveat should be made here, in that not all symptoms associated with a mental health diagnosis can be correlated with neuro-electrical dysregulation. We have observed on countless occasions how symptoms may arise because of other factors. Some symptoms may extend from faulty or harmful cognitions; others from normal processes of grief or bereavement. We will often note relational systems dynamics in which a symptom plays a crucial role in the stabilization of relational patterns, and we routinely screen for medical history to evaluate other variables that can impact symptomology. These symptoms may not present with a neuro-regulatory correlate in the EEG. For this reason, diagnostic processes need to go beyond the analysis of neuro-electrical patterns, utilizing traditional therapeutic, psychiatric, and even medical screens to engage in symptom differentiation.

Even so, the realization that mental health symptomology is frequently related to dysregulation in neuro-electrical patterns is something of a breakthrough for mental health treatment. Analysis of the brain's neuro-electrical activity in light of normative ranges and EEG wave morphology is called a QEEG (Quantitative Electroencephalogram). This powerful assessment tool has consistently demonstrated reliability and validity when compared to tools such as CAT, PET, SPECT, MRI, and fMRI scans. In the last 40 years, the National Library of Medicine's database has listed over 90,000 QEEG studies; a multitude of QEEG studies have cross-validated electrical neuroimaging with the use of structural and functional MRI as well as diffusion spectral imaging to demonstrate the validity of the QEEG to link a person's symptoms to specific brain deviations (Thatcher, 2011). QEEGs are distinctive in that they are able to view EEG baseline patterns over time and assess those patterns according to a normative database for neuro-electrical function. An effective QEEG analysis involves use of research-grade amplifiers that acquire a full 19-channel (or more) recording of EEG over the course of a 5–10 minute baseline in both Eyes Open and Eyes Closed conditions. Acquisition should be performed by a Certified Clinician and/or Technician who is trained to recognize avoidable artifacts in the EEG and obtain impedance levels below 5 k Ohms. Task conditions may or may not be necessary and are evaluated on a person-by-person basis. QEEGs acquired by 2-or 4-channel systems should be avoided, as this is similar to trying to splice together a panorama with 5 or 6 different pictures. The current trend is moving towards automated assessment through algorithm-based software. This is helpful but presents a far from accurate assessment. In the end, the best QEEG analysis is done by a QEEG Diplomate who is trained to analyze the raw EEG data and complete the analysis using multiple montages and databases through a versatile EEG software tool. The report should identify key characteristics of the EEG along with a summary of significant findings and recommendations for training protocols. An effective QEEG analysis can provide unparalleled diagnostic insight into the nature and neurophysiological root of the symptoms associated with mental health disorders. QEEGs are also able to identify brain injury and trauma; they can correlate with many somatizations (such as sleep disorders, chronic headaches, stimming behaviors, or irritable bowel syndrome); and they can guide medication prescribers in the selection of the right medication according to EEG presentation.

The usefulness and functionality of the QEEG is significant enough to warrant a change in basic assumptions about the way we diagnose mental health pathology. Not only is it possible to diagnose anxiety, but with the QEEG we now know that there are at least seven or eight different ways the human brain might dysregulate and still produce a DSM-V diagnosis of GAD. OCD develops from at least three different dysregulations. The traumatized brain is a far more complex condition than the embarrassingly limited diagnosis of PTSD can possibly detail. The myriad of symptoms associated with ADHD—from focus issues to hyperactivity to impulsivity to socializing problems—are easily conceptualized. With the QEEG, we can understand the nature of PDD and see the neuro-electrical underpinnings of ODD, mood instability, and behavioral outbursts. We can identify the markers of Autism, and we can differentiate between a Spectrum disorder versus a dysregulation of brain regions associated with socializing, emotion, and empathy. Effective QEEG analysis allows mental health professionals, for the first time, to assess the functioning of the organ primarily responsible for behavior. For those struggling with mental health issues beyond their ability to contain or control with consistency, this comes as a welcome development, indeed!

Beyond the diagnostic value of QEEG, the important element to note is our ability to change dysregulated brain activity, resulting in remediation of associated symptomology. Effective QEEG analysis generates neurofeedback protocols that target-train dysregulated areas. The more these areas are trained, the more the patterns shift and symptoms resolve. Neurofeedback, then, is a very direct and effective application of neuroplasticity which states that, far from being a static, inflexible organ, the brain is dynamically able to adapt and reorganize itself by forming new neuronal connections throughout life. Neuronal connections form and reinforce through sustained and repeated activation. As it is frequently stated, "neurons that fire together, wire together." Neurofeedback treatment is oriented around this principle, which, in practice, is like training your brain with a neuro-electrical workout. Since neuroplasticity actually enhances neuronal connection on a physiological level, changes that are made and reinforced with neurofeedback are enduring and do not diminish over time.

At The Neurovation Center, we treat PTSD by integrating QEEG analysis, EMDR and other supportive therapeutic models, and neurofeedback training. The treatment of PTSD using neurofeedback was pioneered by Peniston and Kulkosky, who used an alpha/theta protocol to treat 29 combat veterans with PTSD and reported improvements in personality scores and reductions in psychotropic medication use (Peniston and Kulkosky, 1991). Multiple studies since then have replicated these findings. With recent advances in QEEG-guided neurofeedback, we are now able to benefit both from the conventional alpha/theta protocols as well as more individualized and complex protocols (such as z-Score or sLORETA) that target-train the various presentations of nervous system over-arousal associated with trauma. The strength of neurofeedback is in its ability to enhance the individual's focus and concentration, stabilize mood, reduce arousal, and inhibit emotional activity. It is also able to remediate underlying (or phenotypical) EEG characteristics that render an individual more prone to PTSD. EMDR, on the other hand, tends to desensitize the emotional distress associated with traumatic memories. It is a "trigger buster" that allows the individual to gain ownership of their painful memories, not be owned by them. In the end, we like to say that "neurofeedback opens the closet door so that the skeletons can fall out. EMDR cleans up and organizes the bones."

Jeffrey J. Schutz, MA, MA, LMFT, BCN, ORD, is the founder and Executive Director of The Neurovation Center in Sandy Hook, Connecticut. He has authored articles on therapy with special needs populations, spoken at both national and international conferences on Neurofeedback, and provides supervisory training for Neurofeedback clinicians.

Lindsay K. Higdon, MS, QEEG-D, BCN, is the Clinical Director of Neurofeedback Services and Senior QEEG Analyst and Diplomat at The Neurovation Center. Lindsay is expert in the analysis of QEEGs as they are utilized in the Neurofeedback process.

References

Etkin, A., & Wagner, T.D. (2007). "Functional Neuroimaging of Anxiety: A Meta-Analysis of Emotional Processing in PTSD, Social Anxiety Disorder, and Specific Phobia." *American Journal of Psychiatry, 164* (10), 1476–1488.

Lanius, R.A., Frewen, P.A., Tursich, M., Jetly, R., & McKinnon, M.C. (2015). "Restoring Large-Scale Brain Networks in PTSD and Related Disorders: A Proposal for Neuroscientifically-Informed Treatment Interventions." *European Journal of Psychotraumatology, 6*. doi: http://dx.doi.org.proxy1.calsouthern.edu/10.3402/ejpt.v6.27313

Peniston, E.G., & Kulkosky, P.J. (1991). "Alpha-Theta Brainwave Neuro-Feedback Therapy for Vietnam Veterans with Combat Related Post-Traumatic Stress Disorder." *Medical Psychotherapy, 4*, 47–60.

Pole, N. (2007). "The Psychophysiology of Posttraumatic Stress Disorder: A Meta-Analysis." *Psychological Bulletin, 133* (5), 725–746.

Thatcher, R.W. (2011). "Neuropsychiatry and Quantitative EEG in the 21st Century." *Neuropsychiatry, 1* (5), 495–514. doi: http://dx.doi.org.proxy1.calsouthern.edu/10.2217/npy.11.45

Appendix 5
EMDR Case Conceptualization

First name or initials: Age: Gender: M/ F
Occupation:

Presenting problem(s):

1.
2.
3.

Treatment goals:

1.
2.
3.

Genogram showing parents, siblings, and any children, and relationship type/ strength with each (can do narrative if don't know how to draw genogram):

What this suggests about the client's attachment style to you and others:
Secure   Avoidant   Preoccupied   Disorganized

Strengths (support system, faith, hobbies):

Trauma history:

1.
2.
3.
4.

Type of case:

Single event   Single issue with multiple incidents   Multiple issue complex trauma
   Explain your choice:

Intervention plan:

1. Need for resource development? What kinds of resource are needed?

2. Initial target(s)

(Accessed from personal communication in 2015)

Helen Stoller, Psy.D., L.P., approved EMDR consultant. She began work as a licensed psychologist in 1995. She is the director of Psychological and Counseling Associates of the Lowcountry in Bluffton, South Carolina.

Appendix 6
Progressive Muscle Relaxation Technique

1. Tense and relax each muscle group twice before proceeding to the next muscle group. Movement of relaxation is up the body, like a wave.
2. Start with your feet. Notice how they feel in their resting state. Tense your feet by curving your toes toward your heels, as if you were trying to hold onto a tree branch with your feet. Hold the tension as you breathe deeply in through your nose and out through your mouth several times. Release the tension abruptly and notice the tension draining out of your feet. (Noticing, tensing while breathing, relaxing while noticing is the pattern to follow for each muscle group described in the following instructions. Remember to do each muscle group twice.)
3. Move up to your ankles and calf muscles. Tense them by pulling your toes forward toward your shins. You should feel this in your ankles, calves, and shins.
4. For the thigh muscles, tighten them by pulling them together as if to squash a rubber ball between them. You might notice tension in your buttocks as you do this.
5. Pull the abdomen down and toward your buttocks while pulling the buttocks forward and up toward the stomach.
6. Take stock of how your body feels at this point. Hopefully, the lower half of your body is feeling heavy, warm, and relaxed.
7. Move up to your chest. Tighten your chest muscles by pulling your shoulders forward and down, curving your chest wall in toward your back.
8. Tighten your back muscles by pulling your shoulder blades together, which pushes your chest out. **DON'T DO THIS PART if you have any lower back pain.**
9. Tighten your hands and arms by making your hands into fists and curling them up toward your chest as if you were lifting barbells up to your chest. You might find that your hands shake from the tension.
10. Hunch your shoulders up toward your ears.
11. For the face and neck, pull your chin down toward your chest, purse your mouth into a grimace, pull your nose up toward your eyes, and squeeze your eyes together to make your face into a tight, grimacing mask.

12. Notice how heavy, warm, and relaxed your body feels. You might feel somewhat lightheaded at this point.
13. If you wish, you can use visual imagery at this point (imagining with all of your senses a calm, relaxing, safe place) to increase the mental and emotional relaxation you feel.

Helen Stoller, Psy.D., L.P. (2000) approved EMDR consultant (Accessed from personal communication, 2015).

Appendix 7
"Feeding Your Demons"

Feeding your demons rather than fighting them contradicts the conventional approach of fighting against whatever assails us. But it turns out to be a remarkably effective path to inner integration.

Demons (*maras* in Sanskrit) are not bloodthirsty ghouls waiting for us in dark corners. Demons are within us. They are energies we experience every day, such as fear, illness, depression, anxiety, trauma, relationship difficulties, and addiction.

Anything that drains our energy and blocks us from being completely awake is a demon. The approach of giving form to these inner forces and feeding them, rather than struggling against them, was originally articulated by an eleventh-century female Tibetan Buddhist teacher named Machig Labdron (1055–1145). The spiritual practice she developed was called *Chod*, and it generated such amazing results that it became very popular, spreading widely throughout Tibet and beyond.

In today's world, we suffer from record levels of inner and outer struggle. We find ourselves even more polarized, inwardly and outwardly. We need a new paradigm, a fresh approach to conflict. Machig's strategy of nurturing rather than battling our inner and outer enemies offers a revolutionary path to resolve conflict and leads to psychological integration and inner peace.

The method that I have developed, called Feeding Your Demons™, is based on the principles of Chod adapted for the Western world. Here is an abbreviated version of the practice.

5 Steps of Feeding Your Demons

Step 1: Find the Demon in Your Body

After generating a heartfelt motivation to practice for the benefit of yourself and all beings, decide which demon you want to work with. Choose something that feels like it is draining your energy right now. If it's a relationship issue, work the feeling that is arising in you in the relationship as the demon, rather than the other person.

Thinking about the demon you have chosen to work with, perhaps remembering a particular incident when it came up strongly, scan your body and ask yourself: *Where is the demon held in my body most strongly? What is its shape? What is its color? What is its texture? What is its temperature?*

Now intensify this sensation.

Step 2: Personify the Demon

Allow this sensation, with its color, texture, and temperature, to move out of your body and become personified in front of you as a being with limbs, a face, eyes, and so on.

Notice the following about the demon: *size, color, surface of its body, density, gender, if it has one, its character, its emotional state, the look in its eyes, something about the demon you did not see before.*

Now ask the demon the following questions: *What do you want? What do you really need? How will you feel when you get what you really need?*

Step 3: Become the Demon

Switch places, keeping your eyes closed as much as possible. Take a moment to settle into the demon's body. Feel what it's like to be the demon. Notice how your normal self looks from the demon's point of view. Answer these questions, speaking as the demon: *What I want is. . . . What I really need is. . . . When I get what I really need, I will feel . . .* (Take particular note of this answer.)

Step 4: Feed the Demon and Meet the Ally

Take a moment to settle back into your own body. See the demon opposite you. Then dissolve your own body into nectar. The nectar has the quality of the feeling that the demon would have when it gets what it really needs (i.e., the answer to the third question). Notice the color of the nectar.

Imagine this nectar is moving toward the demon and nurturing it. Notice how the demon takes it in. You have an infinite supply of nectar. Feed the demon to its complete satisfaction and notice how it transforms in the process. This can take some time.

Notice if there is a being present after the demon is completely satisfied. If there is a being present, ask it: "Are you the ally?" If it is, you will work with that being. If there is not, or if there is no being present after feeding the demon to complete satisfaction, invite the ally to appear.

When you see the ally, notice all the details of the ally: *size, color, surface of its body, density, gender (if it has one), its character, its emotional state, the look in its eyes, something about the ally you did not see before.*

When you really feel connected with the energy of the ally, ask these questions: *How will you help me? How will you protect me? What pledge do you make to me? How can I access you?*

Change places and become the ally. Take a moment to settle into the ally's body and notice how it feels to be in the ally's body. How does your normal self look from the ally's point of view? When you are ready, answer these questions, speaking as the ally: *I will help you by . . . I will protect you by . . . I pledge I will . . . You can access me by . . .*

Take a moment to settle back into your own body and see the ally in front of you. Look into its eyes and feel its energy pouring into your body.

Now imagine that the ally dissolves into light. Notice the color of this light. Feel it dissolving into you and integrate this luminosity into every cell of your body. Take note of the feeling of the integrated energy of the ally in your body. Now you, with the integrated energy of the ally, also dissolve.

Step 5: Rest in Awareness

Rest in whatever state is present after the dissolution. Pause until discursive thoughts begin again, then gradually come back to your own body. As you open your eyes, maintain the feeling of the energy of the ally in your body.

Allione, L.T. (2016). "Feeding Your Demons." *Lion's Roar, 1* (4), Published Boulder, CO, 33–35 [Reprinted with permission].

Lama Tsultrim Allione is founder and resident lama of Tara Mandala. Ordained as a Buddhist nun at the age of 22, she is the author of two books, *Women in Wisdom* and *Feeding Your Demons*.

Index

Page numbers in italic indicate a figure on the corresponding page.

acupuncture 5
Adaptive Information Processing (AIP) 36, 46–48, 70, 78, 95
Addiction Hope 15–16, 17
Adult Attachment Interview (AAI) 69, 70
Advanced TAC/Audi Scan 48
After the Crash: Psychological Assessment and Treatment of Survivors of Motor Vehicle Accidents 16
Ahmad, Abdulbaghi 37
AIDS 17
akathisia 29
alcoholism 17
Allione, Lama Tsultrim 80
Amann, Benedict L. 39
ambivalent attachment 71
American Foundation for Suicide Prevention 16
American Journal of Psychiatry 25
American Psychiatric Association (APA) 4, 23
American Psychological Association 16, 46
Anderssen, Erin 23
"Antidepressants on Trial: Are They a Wonder or a Danger?" 29
anxiety 29, 89
Artigas, Lucina 43, 44
Ativan 29
"Attachment, Anxiety, Internal Working Models" 70
attachment styles 70–73
attention-deficit hyperactivity disorder (ADHD) 1, 89
attunement 80, 108–109
autonomy 67
avoidant attachment 71

balance and harmony 100
Bardin, Anita 86
Beck's Anxiety Inventory (BAI) 41, 64, 90
Beck's Depression Inventory (BDI) 36–37, 39, 41, 64, 90
benzodiazepines 29
Bergmann, Uri 56
"Bessel van der Kolk on Trauma, Development and Healing" 23, 57
bilateral stimulation (BLS) 48, 49
Bini, Lucio 58
BioLateral Sound CD's 59
biopsychosocial system, six constraints in 95–98
bipolar disorder 39–40, 69–70
Blanchard, Edward 16
Blaustein, Margaret 104, 116
blood pressure medications 30
blueprint for therapy, Metaframeworks perspective and 105–108
Body Keeps the Score: Brain, Mind and the Body in the Healing of Trauma, The 25, 28, 46, 55, 57, 66, 84
body scans 49
borderline personality disorder (BPD) 27, 36, 41–42; attachment styles and 71
Bowen Family Systems therapy 7, 67, 68
Bowlby, John 6, 72
brainspotting 58–59
brain stimulating techniques, other 57–58
Breggin, Peter 29
Breunlin, D. 95–97, 99–104, 106, 107

142 Index

Brief Accessibility Responsiveness and Engagement Scale (BARE) 90
Briere, John 66
Brown, Susan 42
"Buddha's Brain: Neuroplasticity and Mindfulness" 76
Buddhism 75–77
Bullard, David 23, 27
Burke, Theresa 26

Calabrese, Joseph F. 69
Calhoun, Patrick S. 65
California Evidence-based Clearinghouse for Child Welfare 46
"Can Tainted Treatment Make a Shock Return?" 58
"Can We Really Tap Our Problems Away? A Critical Analysis of Thought Field Therapy" 59
Carlat, Daniel 30–31
Carlson, Eve Bernstein 69
case conceptualization, EMDR 4, 6, 11, 33, 35, 93, 134–135
Center for Behavioral Health Statistics and Quality 17, 46
Center for Self-Leadership 73
Centers for Disease Control and Prevention 46
Cerletti, Ugo 58
childhood trauma 12–14; EMDR for 37–38
Clinician-Administered PTSD Scale for Adults (CAPS) 64, 65, 91
Cognitive Behavioral Theory (CBT) 5, 27–28
Colelli, Gina 40
"Color Coded Timeline Trauma Genogram, The" 68
combat-related stress disorders 17, 42–43
"Comparison of Two Treatments for Traumatic Stress: A Community-Based Study of EMDR and Prolonged Exposure" 36
complex trauma 12–15
"Complex Trauma in Children and Adolescents" 104
Conjoint Family Therapy 86
Contextual Therapy 7
continuum of care 43–44
conversing 106–107
Cook, Alexandra 104
COPE Inventory 69, 70

Couple Adaptation to Traumatic Stress Model (CATS) 14–15
Couples Satisfaction Scale Index (CSI-16) 90
"Creating Healing Relationships for Couples Dealing With Trauma: The Use of Emotionally Focused Marital Therapy" 84
Crest 46

Davidson, Richard J. 76
debriefing 51
Delaney, Eileen 24
Depakote 29
DESNOS (Disorders of Extreme Stress Not Otherwise Specified) 12
de Zulueta, Felicity 71
"Diagnostic Accuracy of the PTSD Checklist: A Critical Review, The" 65
Diagnostic Interview for Children and Adolescents (DICA) 38
diagnostic tools 64–70
"Disorders of Extreme Distress: The Empirical Foundation of a complex Adaptation to Trauma" 15
"Disorders of Extreme Stress: The Empirical Foundation of a Complex Adaptation to Trauma" 23
disorganized attachment 71
dissociation 55, 66
Dissociative Experience Scale (DES) 37, 64, 69–70, 91
Doblin, Rick 30
Drozd, John F. 56
DSM-V *(Diagnostic and Statistical Manual of Mental Disorders)* 22–26, 28, 65, 91

"Early EMDR Intervention Following a Community Critical Incident: A Randomized Clinical Trial" 44
Ecstasy 30
Effexor 29
electroconvulsive therapy (ECT) 5, 58
electroencephalogram (EEG) 130–132; biofeedback 130
EMDR (Eye Movement Desensitization and Reprocessing): bipolar disorder and 69–70; borderline personality disorder and 41–42; case conceptualization 4, 6, 11, 33, 35, 93, 134–135; for children 37–38; clinical implications of 114;

Index 143

combat-related stress disorders and 42–43; compared to CBT 28; core components of 46–52; defined 35–36; discovery of 4, 33; efficacy of 38–40; evidence-based practices 4–5, 35–46; Family Systems Therapy integrated with 84–93; following terrorism 40–41; future research on 115–118; genograms in 6, 38, 67–69, 91; holistic approach 5–6; intake, screening, and diagnostic tools 64–70; as integrated approach 5; Internal Family Systems (IFS) and 6, 55, 64, 66–67, 73–75, 83–84; Metaframeworks perspective 6–7, 83–109; mindfulness and 6, 59–60, 66, 75–81; neurobiological components of 34; overview of phases of 125–126; phase eight 51–52; phase five 49; phase four 48–49; phase one 48; phase seven 51; phase six 49; phase three 48; phase two 48; polyvagal theory and 6, 49–51; practical implications of integration of 8; Shapiro on 4, 28, 33–34, 35–36; Stickgold on 34–35; summary of 112–114; therapist role 52–61, 114–115

"EMDR, Adaptive Information Processing and Case Conceptualization" 4, 33–34, 35–36

"EMDR: A Putative Neurobiological Mechanism of Action" 34

EMDR as an Integrated Psychotherapy Approach: Experts of Diverse Orientations Explore the Paradigm Prism 46

EMDR International Association (EMDRIA) 35, 41, 53, 59

"EMDR in Conjunction with Family Systems Therapy" 87

"EMDR Protocol for Recent Critical Incidents [EMDR-PREDI]: Application in a Disaster Mental Health Continuum of Care Context, The" 43

"EMDR's Neurobiological Mechanisms of Action: On the Survey of 20 Years of Searching" 56

"EMDR Therapy Following the 9/11 Terrorist Attacks: A Community-Based Intervention Project in New York City" 40–41

"EMDR Treatment for Children with PTSD: Results of a Randomized Controlled Trial" 37

"EMDR within a Family Systems Perspective" 86

Emotional Freedom Techniques (EFT) 59

Emotionally Focused Therapy (EFT) 84–85

Engler, Jack 73–74

"Enhancing Attachments: Conjoint Couple Theory" 72

"Epidemiology of the Relationship between Traumatic Experience and Suicidal Behaviors" 16

evidence-based practices in EMDR 4–5, 35–46

Experiential Therapy 7

"Expert Answers on E.M.D.R." 53

"Eye Movement Desensitization and Reprocessing in Subsyndromal Bipolar Patients with a History of Traumatic Events: A Randomized, Controlled Pilot-Study" 39, 70

"Family Genogram Interview: Reliability and Validity of a New Interview Protocol, The" 68–69

Family Systems Therapy (FST) 84–93, 114, 117

FDA (Food and Drug Administration) 28–29, 30, 58

"FDA Warns that Paxil Makes Depressed Adults Suicidal" 29

Feeding Your Demons: Ancient Wisdom for Resolving Inner Conflict 81, 138–140

Fernandez, Isabel 39

"Five Things You Should Know About the New DSM Mental-Health Bible" 23

Flynn, Laurie 69

free will 54

Freund, B. 36

"From DSM-IV-TR to DSM-V: Changes in Posttraumatic Stress Disorder" 24

Garcia, Francisca 39

Gaudiano, Brandon A. 59

Geertz, Clifford 5

Generalized Anxiety Disorder 1

genograms 6, 38, 67–69, 91

144 Index

Germer, Christopher 75
GlaxoSmithKline (GSK) 29
Godbout, Natacha 66
Goff, B. S. 14
Grand, David 58–59

Hamzelou, Jessica 17, 18, 58
Handbook of EMDR and Family Therapy Processes, The 85
Harper, Melvin L. 56
Harvard Traumatic Questionnaire (HTQ) 65
Harvard-Uppsala Trauma Questionnaire for Children (HUTQ-C) 38
"Healing from Trauma: Utilizing Effective Assessment Strategies to Develop Accessible and Inclusive Goals" 64
Herbert, James D. 59
Herbine-Blank, Toni 83–84, 101
Herman, Judith Lewis 12–13
Higdon, Lindsay K. 57
Hirschfeld, Robert M. A. 69–70
Hodges, Monica 66
Holmes, Jeremy 71, 72
Houston, Ashley A. 24–25
"How Trauma Impacts the Brain" 26
Husney, Adam 29
hypothesizing 106

Impact of Event Scale-Revised (IES-R) 41, 65, 91
In an Unspoken Voice: How the Body Releases Trauma and Restores Goodness 11, 25, 52, 66, 72, 75
"Inducing Traumatic Attachment in Adults with a History of Child Abuse: Forensic Applications" 71
insecure attachments 71
intake 64–70
"Integrated Neurobiology Approach to Psychotherapy, An" 3
Integrated Problem-Centered Therapy: A Synthesis of Family, Individual and Biological Therapies 90, 96, 100
integrated thinking 14
"Integrating IFS with Phase-Oriented Treatment of Clients with Dissociative Disorder" 66
Integrative Family Therapy 7
Integrative Problem-Centered Therapy: A Synthesis of Family, Individual, and Biological Therapies 96

Internal Family Systems (IFS) model 6, 55, 64, 66, 73–75, 83–84; *see also* Metaframeworks perspective
International Classification of Diseases (ICD) 22–23
International Practice Guidelines for Post-trauma Mental Health (ISTSS) 118
International Society of Traumatic Stress Studies 4
interpersonal effects of trauma 14–15
"Interpersonal Neurobiology Approach to Psychotherapy, An" 77
"Introduction to IFS, An" 73
Ironson, G. 36

Janet, Pierre 66, 112
Jarrero, Ignacio 43, 44
Jeffreys, Matt 28
John Bowlby and Attachment Theory 71
Johnson, Susan M. 84–85
Jordan, Karin 68
Jung, Carl 8

Kabat-Zinn, Jon 6, 76
Kanewischer, Erica J. W. 114–115
Kaslow, Florence W. 85, 87, 88
Keck, Paul E. 69–70
Klonopin 29
Knipe, James 40
Knox, Kerry L. 16
Kramer, Gregory 79

Labdron, Machig 81
Lamictal 29
Landin-Romero, Ramon 39
Lane, Christopher 23
Larsson, Bo 37
Laub, Brurit 44–46
Levine, Peter 2–3, 52; on attachment issues 72; on diagnosis of trauma 25–26; on spirituality 75; on torment of traumatic memories 10–12, 111
Lewis, Lydia 69
Lexapro 29
Life Events Checklist for DSM-V (LEC) 64
"Limits of Talk: Bessel van der Kolk Wants to Transform the Treatment of Trauma, The" 57
Luber, Marilyn 43
Lutz, Antoine 76

Mac Kune-Karrer, B. 106
Major Depression 1
Man and His Symbols 8
mandala 7–8, 112
Mate, Gabor 52
Mayo Clinic 60
Maxfield, Louise 85, 88
McDonald, Scott D. 65
McKenna, Peter J. 39
MDMA 30
Medicaid 23
Medicare 23
medications 28–31
Metaframeworks: Transcending the Models of Family Therapy 99
Metaframeworks perspective 6–7, 93–95, 114, 117; blueprint for therapy 105–108; Family Systems Therapy and 84–93; mindfulness and 108–109; six constraints in the biopsychosocial system and six constraints within 95–96; six constraints within 98–105; web of constraints in 94
mindfulness 6, 59–60, 66, 75–81, 108–109
"Mindfulness: What Is It? What Does It Matter?" 75
Mindfulness of Psychotherapy, The 75
Mindful Therapist: A Clinician's Guide to Mindsight and Neural Integration, The 80, 108–109
Mindsight: The New Science of Personal Transformation 70
minor depression 89
"Mirror Neuron-Mindfulness Hypothesis" 80
Mood Disorder Questionnaire (MDQ) 69–70
mood stabilizing medications 29
Moses, Mark D. 72
motor vehicle accidents 16

National Association of State Mental Health Program Directors 23
National Center for PTSD 1, 16, 28, 29, 46
National Child Traumatic Stress Network (NCTSN) 12–13, 46, 69, 73, 104
National Comorbidity Survey 15
National Criminal Justice Reference Service 46
National Institute for Health and Care Excellence (UK) 58

National Institute of Health (NIH) 22
National Institute of Mental Health (NIMH) 23, 29, 46
National Institute on Alcohol Abuse and Alcoholism 17, 46
National Registry for Evidence-based Programs and Practices 46
"Natural Flow EMDR" 59
Naval Center for Combat & Operational Stress Control (NCCOSC) 24
negative cognitions (NC) 48, 127–128
"Neurobiology of Childhood Trauma and Abuse, The" 13, 48, 54–55
neuroception 50, 60, 72
neurofeedback 57, 129–133
neuroplasticity 59, 75–76, 114–115
Neuro-Tack Corporation 48
Neurovation Center 6, 57, 130, 132
Neustifter, Ruth C. 1, 2
Newmann, Katinka Blackford 29
New Scientist 17, 18, 29
New York Times 28, 53
nightmares 29
Novo, Patricia 39
NPR Fresh Air Interview: Psychiatrist Daniel Carlat 30
Nurse, A. Rodney 87

"On the Neural Base of EMDR Therapy: Insights from (qEEG) Studies" 56

Paxil 28–29
Pelcovitz, David 15, 23
perspectivism 95, 116
Pinsof, W. M. 96, 100
planning/relating 106
Platt, Lisa F. 68–69
polyvagal theory 6, 49–51, 52–53, 59; mindfulness and 77
Polyvagal Theory, The 6, 49–51, 52–53, 60, 77
Pomarol-Clotet, Edith 39
Poole, A. Desmond 88
Porges, Stephen W. 6, 49–51, 52–53, 59, 60; on mindfulness 77
positive cognitions 127–128
Post, Robert M. 69
Post-Traumatic Stress Disorder (PTSD) 10; assessment tools 64–65; borderline personality disorder and 27, 39–40; comorbid mental health diagnoses 15; due to motor vehicle

accidents 16; factors in susceptibility to developing 18; prevalence of 1, 3; role of neurofeedback in treating 129–133; suicide and 16; veterans with 17
Post Traumatic Stress Disorder Symptom Scale (PSS-SR) 36
Posttraumatic Stress Disorder Symptom Scale—Self-Report Version (PSS-SR-17) 65
"Posttraumatic Stress Disorder Treatment Outcome Research: The Study of Unrepresentative Samples" 116
Posttraumatic Stress Symptom Scale for Children (PTSS-C Scale) 38
post-traumatic syndrome 12–13
power: perspectivism and 95; resilience and 2
"Power, Agency, and Resilience after Trauma" 1
Prazosin 29
"Prazosin for PTSD" 29
presence 80, 108–109
Progressive Muscle Relaxation Technique 6, 136–137
protocol, EMDR: exploring attachment styles in 70–73; intake, screening, and diagnostic tools 64–70; Internal Family Systems (IFS) in 73–75; mindfulness in 75–81
Prozac 28
PsychCentral 28–29
"Psychiatrist Daniel Carlat-A Psychiatrist's Prescription for his Profession" 30
Psychology Today 23
psychotherapy.net 23, 27, 57
Psychotherapy Networker 27, 57
PTSD Checklist-Civilian Version (PCL-C) 64, 65, 91
PTSD Checklist-Military Version (PCL-M) 64, 65
PTSD Symptom Scale-Self-Report Version (PSS-SR-17) 65
Putnam, Frank W. 69

Quantitative Electroencephalogram (QEEG) 56, 131–133

Raboni, Mara Regina 38–39
Radua, Joaquim 39
Rasolkhani-Kalhorn, Tasha 56
reading feedback 107

reconsolidation therapy 30
re-evaluation 51–52
Religion as a Cultural System 5
Remeron 29
resilience and power 2
resonance 80, 108–109
Rogers, Susan 40
Roth, Susan 15, 23
Russell, Mark C. 42–43

Sachs, Gary S. 69
Sandy Hook school shooting 8–9, 41, 113, 121–124
Schutz, Jeffrey J. 57
Schwartz, Arielle 50, 51
Schwartz, Richard C. 73, 106
screening 64–70
"Self in Relationship: An Introduction to IFS Couple Therapy" 83, 101
Shapiro, Elan 44, 45–46
Shapiro, Francine 4, 28, 39, 42; Adaptive Information Processing model 46–48, 70, 95; on benefits of integrating EMDR with Family Systems Therapy 85; on bilateral stimulation 48; discovery of EMDR 33–36; on EMDR for community critical incidents 44–46; on practical role of the EMDR therapist 53
Shellenberger, Sylvia 67
Sherman, M. D. 14
Siegel, Daniel J. 3, 70, 77, 79–80, 108–109
Siegel, Irene 59–60
Siegel, Ronald 77
Silver, Steven 40–41
Skeptical Inquirer 59
Smith, D. B. 14
Smith, Tracy K. 1
Smyth, Nancy J. 88
Spinazzola, Joseph 15, 23, 104, 116
Spitzer, Robert L. 69
SSRIs 28
"SSRIs for PTSD: Just How Effective Are They?" 28
Stickgold, Robert 34–35
Stoller, Helene 93
Strauss, J. L. 36
Stressful Life Events Screening Questionnaire (SLESQ) 64–65
Structural Clinical Interview 90
Structural Family Therapy 7
Subjective Units of Distress (SUD) 38, 42, 49, 60

Subjective Units of Disturbance Scale (SUD) 41
Substance Abuse and Mental Health Services Administration 4
Substance Abuse and Mental Health Services Administration (SAMHSA) National Registry for Evidence-based Programs and Practices 46
Suchecki, Deborah 38
suicide 3, 16; antidepressants and 29
"Suicide: 2016 Facts and Figures" 16
Sunday, Susanne 15, 23
Sundelin-Wahlsten, Viveka 37
Surry, Janet L. 79
systemic thinking 14

talk therapy 26–28
tapping/energy psychology (EFT) 5
Tegretol 29
terrorism 40–41
theory of constraints 94
therapists, EMDR 52–61, 114–115
Thompson, Peggy 87
Topimax 29
Torres, Anibal Bernal 64
"Toward a Theory of Constraints" 96, 100
tracking 107
Transcranial Magnetic Stimulation (TMS) 60
"Transcranial Magnetic Stimulation for the Treatment of Adults with PTSD, GAD, or Depression: A Review of Clinical Effectiveness and Guidelines" 60–61
trauma: attachment styles and 70–73; beauty in healing of 111–112; as cause of suicide 3; childhood survivors of 12–14; comorbid mental health diagnoses 15; complex 12–15; definition of 1; dissociation in 55, 66; early research on 10–11; impact of 2; interpersonal effects of 14–15; manifestation of 1–2, 12; medication not healing pervasive 28–31; power and resistance role in defining experience with 2; preparing future practitioners for treating 114–115; prevalence of 3; staggering statistics on 15–19; talk therapy as insufficient for 26–28; violence as source of 17, 18–19, 121–124; warfare as source of 17; world of 68, 69

Trauma and Memory: Brain and Body in a Search for the Living Past 2, 10, 111
"Trauma Causes, Statistics, Signs, Symptoms and Side-effects" 17
Traumatic History Questionnaire (THQ) 64–65, 91
Traumatic Life Events Questionnaire (TLEQ) 64
"Traumatic Stress, Affect Dysregulation, and Dysfunctional Avoidance: A Structural Equation Model" 66
"Treating Attachment Issues through EMDR and a Family Systems Approach" 86
"Treating Combat-Related Stress Disorders: A Multiple Case Study Utilizing Eye Movement Desensitization and Reprocessing (EMDR) with Battlefield Casualties from the Iraqi War" 42
"Treatment of PTSD by Eye Movement Desensitization Reprocessing (EMDR) Improves Sleep Quality, Quality of Life, and Perception of Stress" 38
Tufik, Segio 38
Twombly, Joanne H. 66–67

United Kingdom Department of Health 46
United Kingdom National Institute for Health and Care Excellence 58
U.S. Department of Defense 4, 46
U.S. Department of Health and Human Services 46
U.S. Department of Veterans Affairs 4, 46
"Use of the Genogram with Families for Assessment and Treatment" 67
US Food and Drug Administration (FDA) 28, 29, 30, 58
U.S. National Comorbidity Survey Replication 16

Validity of Cognition Scale (VOC) 41
Validity of Positive Cognition (VOC) 38
Validity of the positive Cognition (VOC) 49
Valium 29
van der Kolk, Bessel A. 46, 96–97, 104, 116; on childhood trauma 13–14, 48, 54–55; on cognitive behavioral therapy 27; on complex adaptation to trauma 15, 23–24; on imprint of trauma 26; on SSRIs 28; on trauma

inadequately accounted for in the DSM-V 25
veterans 17, 42–43
"Veterans Fail to Seek Care for PTSD" 17
Vicens, Victor 39
violence as source of trauma 17, 18–19, 121–124

warfare 17
Webb-Murphey, Jennifer 24
WebMD 29
web of constraints *94*
Wesselmann, Debra 86
Wherever You Go, There You Are: Meditation in Everyday Life 6, 76

Whitaker, Robert 29
Wilk, Karen 121
Williams, J. 36
Williams, Janet 69
Williams-Keeler, Lyn 84–85
World Health Organization (WHO) 3, 4, 17, 22, 46
world of trauma 68, 69
Wylie, Mary Sykes 27, 57

Xanax 29

yoga 6, 77

Zajecka, John M. 69
Zoloft 28–29